Cost-Effective Laboratory Management

D1537189

Cost-Effective Laboratory Management

Editor

Paul Bozzo, M.D.
Clinical Professor
Department of Pathology
University of Arizona Health Sciences Center; and
Medical Director
TMCHE Laboratory
Tucson Medical Center
Tucson, Arizona

Foreword by

Brent C. James, M.D., M.Stat.
Vice President for Medical Research and
Executive Director
Intermountain Health Care Institute for
  Health Care Delivery Research
Salt Lake City, Utah

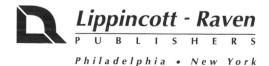

Lippincott - Raven
P U B L I S H E R S
Philadelphia • New York

Acquisitions Editor: Anne S. Patterson
Developmental Editor: Lesa E. Ramsey
Manufacturing Manager: Kevin Watt
Production Manager: Robert Pancotti
Production Editor: Melanie Bennitt
Cover Designer: Joseph DePinho
Indexer: Victoria Boyle
Compositor: Lippincott–Raven Desktop Division
Printer: Maple Vail

Printed in the United States of America

9 8 7 6 5 4 3 2 1

Library of Congress Cataloging-in-Publication Data

Cost-effective laboratory management / editor, Paul Bozzo : foreword
    p. cm.
  Includes bibliographical references and index.
  ISBN 0-397-58773-2
  1. Medical laboratories—Management—Economic aspects. I. Bozzo, Paul, 1938– .
  [DNLM: 1. Laboratories—organization & administration.
2. Laboratories—economics. W 23 C839 1998]
  R860.C67 1998

616.07′56′068—dc21
DNLM/DLC
For Library of Congress
                                      98-21036
                                        CIP

This book is dedicated to those who are struggling with issues of cost, appropriatcness, and people while trying to maintain quality care for the patient as their primary goal.

Contents

Contributing Authors

Paul Bozzo, M.D., *Clinical Professor, Department of Pathology, University of Arizona Health Sciences Center; Medical Director, TMCHE Laboratory, Tucson Medical Center, 5301 East Grant Road, Tucson, Arizona 85712*

Joni S. Condit, M.S., *Vice President of Patient Services, Department of Administration, Tucson Medical Center, 5301 East Grant Road, Tucson, Arizona 85712*

Annette M. Fernandez, M.D., *Global Director of Business Development and Marketing, IgX Ltd., 1 Springfield Avenue, Summit, New Jersey 07901*

C. Martin Harris, M.D., *Chief Information Officer, Chairman of Information Technology Division, The Cleveland Clinic Foundation, 9500 Euclid Avenue, Cleveland, Ohio 44195*

Neil R. Lautaret, M.B.A., *Adjunct Faculty Member, Pima Community College, Tucson, Arizona; Director of Business Operations, Tucson Medical Center Laboratory, 1011 North Craycroft Road, Building 200, Suite 201, Tucson, Arizona 85712*

Rodney S. Markin, M.D., Ph.D., *Professor and Vice Chair, Department of Pathology and Microbiology, Nebraska Health System-University Hospital; Professor and Associate Dean for Clinical Affairs, Department of Pathology and Microbiology, College of Medicine, University of Nebraska Medical Center, 983135 Nebraska Medical Center, Omaha, Nebraska 68198-3135*

William P. Moffitt, B.S., *President and Chief Executive Officer, i-STAT Corporation, 303 College Road East, Princeton, New Jersey 08540*

David B. Nash, M.D., M.B.A., *Associate Dean, Department of Health Policy, Jefferson Medical College; Director, Department of Health Policy and Clinical Outcomes, 1015 Walnut Street, Philadelphia, Pennsylvania 19107*

Nancy R. Ryan, B.S., *Marketing Developmental Manager, i-STAT Corporation, 303 College Road East, Princeton, New Jersey 08540*

Foreword

Before 1900, craft-based production created essentially all goods and services that human beings consumed. A skilled craftsman, assisted by apprentices who learned as they worked, handcrafted each unique, customized item—no two were quite the same. Craft apprenticeships provided most education. Within that training system the vast majority of workers, in America and across the world, were illiterate.

In 1911 Frederick Winslow Taylor published a book describing a new theory of production called Scientific Management (1). Scientific Management found its roots in the idea of *processes*—predefined sequences of standardized steps, analyzed and created by university-trained engineers, by which (often) illiterate workers would use standardized parts to produce goods and services. In essence, the workers became cogs in a machine, with little or no discretion, variation, or opportunity for personal creativity. Taylor's personal catch phrase was "the *one* best way." The first major example of Scientific Management was Henry Ford's assembly lines for his new Model T cars.

Some historians rank Taylor's contributions with those of Freud and Darwin in creating modern society (2). Taylor's methods were so much more efficient in creating goods and services than craft-style production that they quickly swept the world. Within 15 years, process-based production—standardized assembly line manufacturing—had supplanted craft-style production across the entire world. It was a transformation similar in magnitude to the industrial revolution, but taking decades rather than centuries. It did not require new machines so much as it changed the ways in which people used existing machines.

That transition also created the foundation for the American middle class. The new assembly lines not only produced more goods but also provided high-paying jobs that gave the working class the means to obtain those less expensive goods. It produced free time and extra resources that enabled average Americans to reach into areas that before were the distant prerogatives of the moneyed upper classes, such as formal education.

Scientific Management had its own limitations, of course. It tended to treat workers as cogs in machines and greatly contributed to the rise of the labor union movement. But its real limitation was *complexity*: How does one design and manage complex processes for which it is impossible to predetermine every step? That is probably why medicine was one of those few niche areas of craft-style production that survived the onslaught of Scientific Management. To this day, expert medical craftsmen create unique, personalized products for individual patients. Medical apprentices (residents and fellows) still learn the art of clinical practice by the hands-on doing of care delivery, under the direct supervision of a credentialed member of the guild. Given the huge variation, in physiology, disease, resources, and preferences, that individual patients bring to physicians, no other approach is practical. It is impossible to predetermine every step of clinical practice.

Recent advances in process theory, many developed within and uniquely adapted to medical practice, are finally beginning to address the complexity conundrum. Those new process management methods, joined together, form clinical quality improvement. The core idea might be called "appropriate standardization." Using modern information technology, expert clinicians can jointly design standardized care delivery processes that still leave them free to vary and to meet unique patient needs (3): "Vary when you must, but comply with the standard when you can." Standardized subsystems are more reliable, so that physicians waste less time and energy correcting mistakes. They move routine, repetitive tasks (the "scut work" of clinical care) to support personnel, leaving physicians free to concentrate on those portions of a patient's care that require customization—the creative, fun part of medicine that fully exercises a physician's creativity and training. Early evidence suggests that such "appropriate standardization" significantly improves clinical outcomes while reducing the costs of care. It suggests that the key to surviving in a competitive, cost-based medical marketplace is to strengthen the core values and functions of the medical profession. It represents, 100 years later, the arrival of Scientific Management within medical practice, but in a uniquely medical way that reinforces medicine as one of the four original "learned professions."

All change is inherently local. Quality improvement theory expresses that truism in the concept of "fundamental knowledge." That is the idea that the only people who truly understand a process are those individuals who directly operate it, day in and day out. This book makes an important contribution to medical practice because it embodies fundamental knowledge at two levels. First, it was written by clinical pathologists for clinical pathologists. It provides practical, proven solutions to real problems from the perspectives of people who fundamentally understand the challenges and tasks of present-day clinical pathology. Second, the clinical pathologists who wrote this book have fundamental knowledge about improvement. One clear implication of "appropriate standardization" is that health care professionals must begin to work together, at an intellectual level, to write down, test, and implement common processes of care. It is particularly useful if some members of that professional group can contribute hands-on experience in process management, focused within that subset of clinical processes that make up a particular specialty. You hold in your hands the condensed experience of such a group of "quality" medical professionals.

Brent C. James, M.D., M.Stat.
Vice President for Medical Research and Executive Director
Intermountain Health Care Institute for Health Care Delivery Research
Salt Lake City, Utah

REFERENCES

1. Taylor, Frederick Winslow. *The Principles of Scientific Management.* New York, NY: W.W. Norton & Company, Inc., 1967 (original edition: 1911, Harper & Row).
2. Kanegil, Robert. *The One Best Way.* New York, NY: Viking Penguin Books, USA Inc., 1997.
3. James, Brent C. Implementing practice guidelines through clinical quality improvement. *Frontiers of Health Services Management.* 1993;10(1):3-37, 54-56 (Fall).

Preface

Deciding to write a book on cost-effective management is impossible if you are limited to relating only your own personal experiences. Every situation offers its own unique potential for learning. This book relates lessons learned and insight gained by multiple authors with a varied focus in the laboratory.

The health care environment is changing more rapidly than anticipated. The emphasis in the media and in managed care appears to be on cost, and financial analysis is discussed in this book with that in mind. However, quality and appropriate testing are also key elements to cost-effective management, which is defined as "Doing the right thing." This book covers topics that are essential to successful management of any size lab team, including evaluations (promoting and hiring the right people is a key to success) and leadership. In addition, effective communication and accuracy require efficient computers and an understanding of the role that they must play in the lab of the future. Debatable but worthwhile topics include point of care testing and robotics. The data provided on these topics will be worthwhile to every manager faced with making decisions in these areas. The focus of this book is to provide the experiences of insightful authors going through change, so that you can make decisions more effectively in your own situation.

Acknowledgments

I acknowledge the efforts of the many people who are not listed as authors but have contributed to this book. Every book starts with a nidus, which in this case was the office of Vickie Thaw from Lippincott-Raven Publishers, ably assisted by Rachael Paul. Subsequent developmental assistance was provided by Anne Patterson and Carol Field. I appreciate all of their suggestions and editing. I also applaud the efforts of each of the authors. I am grateful for the proofing and ideas contributed by Jane Barton, Joni Condit, Rod Pasqualy, Kathy Tanner, Fred Bayer, Alan Madison, Niles Robinson, Kevin Johnson, and Lisa Kimber. No book is completed without logistical and typing assistance, which was provided by Heather Campbell, Todd Leuthjohann, Janette Fisher, and Glades Guisinger, Finally, I am grateful to everyone associated with Tucson Medical Center and TMCHE Lab for providing a work environment that is both stimulating and conducive to learning.

Cost-Effective Laboratory Management

Introduction

Paul Bozzo

I can, I am.
(Graffiti on a wall in Watts taken from the movie *Sugar Hill*.)

This book addresses change and quality improvement in health care. It developed out of mistakes made and lessons learned, and focuses on the lab as part of a larger system. Although laboratory costs represent a small percentage of the budget, they affect the entire system significantly. A media-inflamed public has insisted that escalating costs beyond the rate of inflation be controlled. This has resulted in change, but as managed care and integrated health care systems have cut costs, it has also caused the public to question quality.

The laboratory field has changed dramatically. Twenty years ago, labs did not question orders; quality was assumed. Labs were profitable and were neither cost centers nor competitive businesses. Many were highly successful local mom and pop operations. Today competition is intense. Proof of quality is demanded and fees are declining. With rapid advances in medicine, it is the best of times. With the prevailing public opinion that medicine is overpriced, it is also the worst of times. Our challenge is to cut costs without reducing quality.

Quality is essential to a health care system's survival, whether managed care, an integrated delivery system, or a stand-alone lab. Is improvement occurring at the pace required by the present conditions? Are we actively searching for solutions to such issues as restructuring (reengineering), closing of a little-used nursing ward, flexible scheduling to offset down time, or appropriateness of testing? Can we reduce the error rate and waiting time? Do we work in a learning environment? Are we aiming for zero defect or perfection? We may accept less, but we should do so grudgingly and should work constantly for perfection. Effective leadership with support from the top leaders, who are constantly concerned with quality, is absolutely essential.

Words must be credible and must be supported by actions, especially on the part of leaders. Remember that no list of dos and don'ts can encompass the vagaries of the real world. We hit unexpected obstacles and have the bruises to show for it. We hope that sharing our experiences with you will provide insights for your situation.

Some of the problems faced and conclusions reached may be familiar. We all have unique histories that define our individual or corporate character, but we also share similarities, such as the search for "best value": a composite of accuracy, service, and appropriateness at a reasonable cost. How can we take advantage of the advances in communication, informatics, and technology that have changed the state-of-the-art laboratory? Separate chapters on informatics and robotics address such questions.

State-of-the-art laboratory informatics can provide more accurate management data, increase the accuracy of results, and facilitate communication while speeding up the process. Internet communication and grouped mailboxes offer immediate feedback on rapidly changing issues, including diagnostic test results and graphic representation of parameters of care. Implementation requires a commitment to computers, which means a commitment to providing the funds for state-of-the-art hardware, software, and training. The potential benefits include providing physicians with clinical pathways (approaches to diagnostic and/or therapeutic paths or steps to take when addressing similar situations), triggered by admitting diagnosis, and, ultimately, facilitating consensus orders (clinical orders for patient care which are agreed upon by a group of clinicians). The computer of the future must prioritize customer needs before administrative needs.

Customers of health care expect nothing less than perfection; accuracy and quality are assumed. (Who can forget Johnson and Johnson's experience with the contamination of a few bottles of Tylenol, the public outcry, and the immediate response? All bottles of Tylenol had to be removed from the shelves, an expensive solution to retaining customer confidence and keeping the image of quality.) An improvement in the condition of the patient is the gold standard for decision making. Although the lab is one step removed from the patient, accurate and timely testing can improve the patient's condition. Measuring outcomes is the challenge.

Because patient outcomes are complex and are affected by everyone in health care, that measurement is frequently done by the system. It measures not only mortality, morbidity, and cost, but also the patient's quality of life and satisfaction. The lab should be a participant or a leader in providing data to help measure quality outcomes. This may require large groups of similar patients and long-term follow-up. Although many believe these measurements are being done for the regulatory agencies, both individual and large corporate customers will demand such information soon.

It is important to have a goal and a plan in any endeavor. Goals should change, be prioritized, and relate to the mission statement of your system, and they should be communicated frequently. In reviewing options available to our system, groups dominated by physicians, board members, and managers ranked goals. The quality of care easily ranked first. Caring should be evident at all levels of the organization. Evidence of that caring should be visible in our contact with all our customers. That caring should be reflected by your work-specific goals, which relate to care and which should be known by every employee.

We cannot deal with everything at once, but we can select significant processes critical to patient care, based on high volume, high costs, or difficulty of problems. Regulators—who are now asking laboratories to look at quality improvement related to patient outcome—require a laboratory quality assurance plan, but our plans/goals should go beyond satisfying regulators. One area where the laboratory can affect patient care for the better is to ensure that testing is appropriate. We devote a full chapter to this topic and emphasize ways of modifying physician behavior.

We can refine what we are doing and can improve efficiency, but we must also examine what we are doing. Appropriate test utilization is an extremely important issue in cost control. Approximately 80% of the decisions in health care are controlled by clinicians. Clinical pathways, developed to provide a consensus on the best approach to take, affect clinical decisions. Data showing marked variation in the clinical process provide evidence of this uncertainty. To achieve best value we must reduce variation. All patients are unique, but many uncomplicated, clinically similar situations show a high degree of variation in the clinical process. We looked at some examples of uncomplicated myocardial infarction and found the variations in approach to be significant. Everyone agreed that these patients were similar, but getting clinicians to agree on the approach was difficult. Eventually, consensus was reached. The results showed not only significant savings but improved patient outcome.

Change is not easy. It requires dialogue, a common goal, an open mind, flexibility, comprehensible data, and a respected leader to champion it. A word of caution: We must not immediately assume that more is bad and less is good. Some pathways can result in more laboratory testing. The critical question to be answered is, "Does the clinical pathway improve patient care and patient outcome?"

Computer-generated data can easily monitor some aspects of outcome, including length of stay, financial data, mortality, and morbidity. Patient satisfaction requires data that truly reflect the customer's opinion. I reviewed survey data from a large company that reflected a high percentage of user satisfaction. The conclusion of this survey was based on a question with only three potential answers: *below average, average,* or *above average.* The company assumed *average* or *above average* meant "highly acceptable." This survey was done right after the company had entertained a group of managers and offered continuing education on current and future products. Many other levels of users were not represented. This is an example of misleading information from a survey with poor cross-sectional representation, questions composed in a manner that favored a positive result, and timing that favored a positive response. Patient satisfaction must be measured accurately. We cannot always assume that good composition and content of a survey reflect a good cross section of subjects or an unbiased response. Surveys require knowledgeable people to compose, administer, and interpret results.

A quality-oriented environment requires a cooperative attitude between management, physicians, and every on-line employee. Quality is a way of life, not an additional activity. This requires sharing information in a manner that builds trust, and it means allowing every level to interact in the creative portion of your vision. It took me some time to think of quality as a way of life and not an additional activity. People can't help but participate when they have the information. If you don't share it, the reverse may be true. Noninformed employees may even be a source of internal sabotage.

We devote a full chapter to methods of cost analysis and the validity of cost data. Understanding the tools of financial analysis fosters valid cost-saving measures. More important, cost analysis is used to help validate decisions such as equipment, supplies, sendout tests, robotics, reengineering, mergers, and point-of-care testing. Valid cost per unit of service is valuable information if it truly reflects your costs.

There is only so much money for health care; we should all look at triaging or the prioritization of health care dollars. Richard Lamm, the former governor of Colorado, made this point at a Greater Foundation series in Tucson (November 9, 1995). The miracles we are performing (e.g., transplant surgeries) are creating better health care for a select few. But the limited funding necessary to achieve some of the more difficult results has reduced support for education and preventive care. Triaging of funds is critical if we are to improve health care. Preventive medicine is cost-effective, but it must be done intelligently.

For example, the accuracy of pap smears can be improved by expensive computer-driven screening, followed by rescreening of abnormal smears by cytotechnologists. This increases the cost of routine screening and could therefore result in more women receiving fewer pap smears. Many cases of carcinoma or precarcinoma of the cervix occur in women from lower socioeconomic groups dependent upon government-funded cytologic screening. Thus, if the price of screening goes up and the funding stays the same, fewer pap smears could be performed in this population that is more susceptible to cervical cancer. Unfortunately, cytology is a focus for malpractice. This will favor the more expensive approach, which will increase the detection rate slightly on the cervical smears submitted for screening. Is this the most cost-effective use of health care dollars?

In order to cut costs many organizations are merging, assuming that bigger organizations result in greater cost efficiencies. If such mergers result in poor laboratory service or a decrease in accuracy of test results it could impact clinical decisions and resultant quality of care in a negative manner. The lab leverages many clinical decisions which if less than optimal can result in a lower quality of care which is not cost-effective. Poor quality, for example, increased morbidity, costs. Theoretically, eliminating duplication of personnel and equipment in addition to obtaining large-volume discounts with vendors should lower costs, but accuracy of test results and quality of service must be maintained or improved if a merger is to be successful.

Technological changes such as those resulting from robotics can reduce laboratory costs by as much as 50%. Robotics, which is currently in the initial stages of implementation, will have its greatest impact on larger labs. In addition, multichannel instruments and, at times, multiple instruments, interconnected and controlled by a small personal computer, can reduce the number of personnel while improving accuracy.

How many involved with clinical laboratories are still duplicating prothrombin times or activated partial thromboplastin times because of a tradition dating back to the days of less accurate equipment? How many have carefully examined the precision and/or accuracy of their methods? The cost of unnecessary repetition is one thing, but that of doing something wrong is even greater. This includes not only the performance of the test, but the processes preceding and following it. A good example would be the right lab test done on the wrong patient. Such mistakes not only are costly, but often go undetected. Processes must be examined and changed if they are to be improved. Too frequently we err by selecting a common variation (problem) and by not examining the entire process. Most errors are due to poor processes or lack of training, not to an individual or group.

Needs are not the same as wants. Determining needs requires careful listening and observation to perceive significant modifications that may be necessary in the future. For example, in the late 1980s, who would have foreseen the present need for personal computers or the impact of the Internet? Tom Peters provides an example of the success that can result when the provider of a product or service listens to the needs of the marketplace. He describes the advances the Swiss made in the sale of watches once they decided style was just as significant as accuracy (1).

Everyone talks about listening, but listening with an ear to future needs is part of the creative culture we must embrace. It is no longer enough to ask our customers, "How are we doing?" We must also ask, "What do you want now and in the future?" Most can only speak about the present; the future generally requires reading between the lines. Only by listening very carefully and with some vision for the future can you meet customer needs, and meeting customer needs is necessary to survival.

The health care organization that survives will be a learning organization. It's no accident that those organizations that are constantly growing stress the importance of acquiring and using new knowledge. In many organizations, training is a neglected area. New employee orientation generally includes discussions of benefits, salary issues, safety, body substance precautions, and regulatory concerns. However, formal training in coaching, mentoring, creativity, interpersonal relations, and job cross-training is frequently lacking. Cross-training in the lab promotes better understanding and communication. It allows personnel from different departments or sections to better understand the needs of others as a result of performing their role. This is most productive when it occurs on either side of a handoff. An example of a handoff is the courier who hands specimens to the processing department. If the courier worked in processing, he or she has greater empathy for processing's need to have the specimens delivered in a timely fashion to avoid breakdown of red blood cells which can cause erroneous results. Knowledge promotes empathy and cooperation. It is leadership's responsibility to prioritize and make time available for training that fosters organizational and individual growth.

We must periodically take the time to think about where we're going and what we have accomplished. Constantly working without a plan can result in unachieved goals. The process of reviewing where you are and considering your future creates energy, builds a team, and provides efficiencies of operations. We're already so busy that we think only of survival, which can prohibit creative thinking. Leadership must show its commitment to building an efficient and creative organization by providing the time required for creative thinking.

Culture changes are difficult because culture is based on knowledge and beliefs that generate a behavior pattern. For example, in the past, we have thought of the patient and the physician as the ultimate customers. The customer includes internal customers (other employees) and external customers (not only patients but third-party payers, third-party patient family, and third-party patient friends). It takes time and patience to change a culture.

Fear is frequently the biggest obstacle to change. Sometimes participants fear that real creativity may eliminate their jobs. It is also difficult to change something you may have helped create, especially when that change threatens your position. Fear of change is the obstacle we must overcome. This book addresses our experience with fear and its consequences.

If we make processes more efficient (doing it the right way) and more effective (doing the right thing), fewer employees will be required. This is difficult because you're not eliminating a position, you're laying off someone who may support a family. It may be possible to do this by attrition, but when layoffs are inevitable, it's important to make job placement and additional skill development a priority. The more specialized the position eliminated, the more difficult the job placement, for highly trained individuals wish to use the skills they already possess.

We should not forget that many are in the health care industry because they wanted a profession that allowed them to contribute to the care of their fellow human beings. This includes not only patients, but fellow employees as well. As we focus on best value, we must remember the human touch. People remain the most important part of an organization. People need goals and a vision. They also need positive values, including trust, loyalty, and respect. All this must exist in an environment where there are no job guarantees.

We have not always looked at the laboratory as a business concerned with efficiency and effectiveness. The economic crisis faced by medicine has forced organizations to examine effectiveness and efficiencies. The authors of this book share experiences in certain key areas and hope that the information contained here will help our readers move forward positively in this changing environment.

REFERENCE

1. Peters T: *CAP Today* (Oct. 1992):94.

1

Reengineering

Paul Bozzo

> There is nothing more difficult to plan, more doubtful of success, nor more dangerous to manage than the creation of a new order of things.... Whenever his enemies have the ability to attack the innovator they do so with a passion of partisans, while the others defend him sluggishly, so that the innovator and his party like are vulnerable.
>
> *Niccolo Machiavelli, The Prince*

> Whatever you can do
> or dream you can, begin it.
> Boldness has genius, power,
> and magic in it.
>
> *Goethe*

REENGINEERING, OR SHOULD IT BE CALLED RUNNING A BUSINESS?

Reengineering means reworking processes and rethinking how you do business. Our own situation clearly required a radical change. We couldn't continue to do things as we had. Everything we considered pointed to reengineering as a potential solution. In mid-1994 we began the process of reengineering.

The objective was to merge Tucson Medical Center Hospital Laboratory and Tucson Medical Center Health Enterprise (TMCHE) outpatient laboratory. Since 1994 we have spent considerable time working on a merger with labs in Phoenix, a partnership with a large national lab, and a merger with a community lab. At the time of this writing, we have decided against those mergers and partnerships. If we had been successful, the same process of reengineering would have been used, but ought to have been more efficient because of lessons learned in the past. The principles of reengineering, including the decision-making process and the rationale, are similar for all these situations. This chapter describes our experience with laboratory reengineering and discusses them under four headings: "The Rationale for Reengineering," "The Process of Reengineering," "Outcome," and "Lessons Learned." Mike Hammer defines reengineering as "the fundamental rethinking and radical redesign of business processes to bring about a dramatic improvement in performance.... Reengineering is focused at the process level at how a set of tasks are organized into the whole" (1). This is not the same as downsizing or "rightsizing," which may result in immediate cost savings. We were looking for cash savings by changing processes without losing sight of customer satisfaction. It turned out to be a roller coaster ride.

Rationale for Reengineering

We had the largest hospital laboratory in southern Arizona at one location and the largest commercial laboratory in southern Arizona approximately 1 mile away. We knew that testing, equipment, and both technical and management skills were being duplicated at the two sites, which also had two different cultures. The hospital lab was more structured, the commercial one more freewheeling. The hospital staff was used to a stable, bureaucratic format. The commercial staff was used to frequent change and developing new directions and goals. The hospital was experiencing a decrease in business; business at the commercial lab was increasing, and the lab was moving quickly into more managed-care contracts. The organization was undergoing integration, and its employees were increasing from 2,500 to 5,200. The hospital, managed care, home care, assisted living, a mental health hospital, an orthopedic center, a group of 80 physicians, and the Children's Clinics for Rehabilitative Services were all integrated. In addition, three separate large physician groups (primary care) were consolidated for contractual purposes. At the time, we were not only integrating locally but networking with a view to consolidating with a larger system in Phoenix.

Although I would like to report that the rationale for reengineering was quality improvement, the fact is that it was survival. This may not be the ideal motivation, but historically major changes have occurred when situations reach crisis proportions. We were not at the cliff's edge, but we were close. A purpose beyond survival would be in the future, but during the initial stages, we had to change or lose our jobs. Dialogue about quality and the attempt to give meaning to decisions ideally optimizes performance, but the fear of job loss provided the true leverage.

The system had to reduce costs and to position for the future. The lab was to be no exception. This was made extremely clear when we learned of a competitive bid from a national reference laboratory to our system's managed care, which at the time accounted for 50% of our business and was increasing. At the time of this writing, Tucson has one of the higher penetration rates for managed care in the United States and is expected to be nearly 100% by the year 2000. However, even in countries with socialized medicine such as England or Italy, fee for service remains an option that is still used by about 5% of the population. University Health System Consortium has market classifications based on a number of criteria, including managed-care admissions to hospitals, the percentage of total patient population associated with managed care, and physician involvement. Based on these criteria, in 1994 Tucson was a level III consolidation. At the time of this writing, we are level IV consolidation, the highest bracket. As of January 5, 1997, 41% of health care in Tucson is managed care (2) and more than 75% of employers are purchasing managed health care coverage.

Managed care implies health care with fixed financial resources. Perhaps *fixed* is not a good term because, despite inflation, less money is available to the lab than in the past. The competitive nature of managed health care is forcing a flat field financially; presently, price, not quality, appears to be the most important factor. However, employers (buyers) are asking for accountability and demanding outcome data. It appears that for employers, quality is rapidly becoming more of an issue and is not assumed. In addition, there is a greater interest in preventive health services.

If you discuss issues with patients of the laboratory, as I sometimes do, accuracy is not a frequent topic. These customers are concerned with such issues as communication, timely results, how long they have to wait, and the efficiency with which blood is drawn; these govern their perception of laboratory quality. They assume that the test results are accurate.

We must have a global understanding of the economics of the health care environment and understand our customers' future needs (patients, third-party payers, systems), be flexible, and develop a vision with a sound plan; otherwise we may find ourselves out of business. The changes that we are seeing were predictable, but the pace with which they are occurring is much faster than anticipated.

As an example of rapid change, consider our own experience with one of our largest customers, a managed-care company partially owned by our system. The question we faced was, "Can we partner with our managed-care partners?" We had not done a good job of communication and partnering with them in the past, but for communication to occur effectively, we would have to not only be part of their team but to take the lead. The problem was that the managed-care organization owned and sponsored by the system wanted a positive bottom line. Their finances were a matter of public record both locally and statewide, and they felt that a negative bottom line would affect their ability to increase market share. We (the lab) were thus capitated at a rate that was below our costs, and senior leadership dictated where our dollars went. We quickly understood the difficulty of partnering with an organization whose driving force is cost.

We considered an unpredictable future and weighed the risk. If we gave up the managed-care business, we would also give up the associated fee-for-service (discretionary) business that we gained by servicing those private clinical offices, along with large volumes of testing, which gave us better operating efficiencies. Even though the laboratory was owned by the same system that owned the managed-care operation, a task force was organized to review bids for laboratory services. The task force included physicians and administrators from multiple factions of the system including our executive administrator, Joni Condit; Gerry Gilmore, the system vice-president who is responsible for the laboratory; and myself.

I looked around the room and saw people from some outside administrative groups whom I barely knew, along with a group of familiar physicians. We would have to become aligned with the different administrative sources if we wanted to keep this managed-care contract. It felt as if the laboratory was on trial. What had we done or not done to be put in this predicament? Perhaps we hadn't faced reality and had not thought enough about the external environment. I reflected on the past, when physicians had an unrestricted credit card and patients became anemic because so much blood was drawn for diagnostic testing. I, for one, had sat back quietly questioning the amount of testing but did nothing to curb this abuse of laboratory services. In those days we had a different view of efficiency of operation. If the work was not done on a timely basis, then more people were hired. If physicians wanted an unusual test run locally for their convenience, we set it up. It didn't matter that running a small number of tests would not be cost-effective and would require expensive controls for each run. In addition, training for infrequent esoteric tests would add significantly to the cost per test.

The laboratory was a profit center. We did work, we billed enough to make a profit, and we were paid. But even then we listened to our customers, since the physicians' concerns were considered paramount to the lab's success. If they wanted something, they got it. We just charged to cover the cost and built in a profit. If we had grown and matured enough to anticipate the pressures of the managed-care concept, Joni, Gerry, and I might not have been in this meeting. We were not behind most areas of the organization in dealing with change; in fact, we were facing some issues of "best value" sooner than most. Best value was optimizing the combination of service, accuracy, and cost. However, service and accuracy were taken for granted; cost was the true issue. We had some data on service—namely, a few monitors of turnaround time and a large amount of information on accuracy—because laboratories were always involved in strict control of the testing itself. We knew that more problems occur in the ordering and preparation of specimens than in the actual testing.

The customers were many, but the driver was the payer, who was interested only in price. We felt with time the payer would also look at quality. With a facilitator, we brainstormed on the advantages and disadvantages of subcontracting to a major reference laboratory. It was very uncomfortable to hear a discussion of the possibility of closing a commercial laboratory that you had been a part of since its inception and a hospital laboratory that you had worked in for almost 25 years. In reality, the question being asked was, "Is the system laboratory a core value for the system?" This is a frequently used buzzword. A core value is one that presents your system with advantages that would be lost by subcontracting. It represents a value that you would retain and control because it offers some competitive advantage. I felt we were a core value, as did the physicians at that meeting. Interestingly, and not too unexpectedly, the physicians on the task force had a historical perspective of service, accuracy, and leadership, resulting in *some* confidence in our abilities. These areas would have to continue to improve if we were to survive.

This confidence in the positive aspects of the laboratory would be lost if the system went with a national commercial laboratory. If the decision had been to go with a national laboratory, it would be extremely difficult and expensive for us to return later to the present level of service. If the loss of the system laboratory proved unacceptable to its customers, then equipment would have to be brought back from the national lab for a preset amount and the system lab would have to be reestablished in a structured format set forth in the original contract. This would be easier said than done. In our view, the key disadvantage of subcontracting lab services would be loss of control. The physicians on the task force were concerned about this and about having to work with a consultant pathologist whom they did not know or have confidence in. Certain areas—namely, surgical pathology, cytology, and microbiology—received a more positive review. I was surprised that hematology and the pathologist's involvement with abnormal differentials were not a concern. The physicians believed that chemistry tests were done with automated equipment and with the same quality for all labs. No discussion of protesting, quality control, or quality improvement occurred.

An additional issue discussed was appropriate utilization. This was brought up at the time of the meetings, but there was minimal discussion of physician ordering patterns. Managed care showed little concern because the laboratory was only about 1% of its budget, although it would have been a bigger part if they paid for the true cost of testing. Participants appeared unconcerned about the degree to which the lab leveraged other health care provider decisions. Managed care's concept of the laboratory as a unique part of a system that dovetailed smoothly with other areas was not considered. Managed care was concerned about cost but interested in key customer (physician) opinion of the service issues. The role of effective laboratory leadership would include managing interactions within the system. This would be much easier if we were truly part of a system team. The national reference lab had made significant promises to win the business and obviously wanted to position itself for the future, for fewer labs, less competition, and therefore hoping for more freedom to increase prices.

The final decision of the task force, including a strong physician vote, was to support the laboratory as a core value for the system. The message was loud and clear: *Get the cost down and give us the same or better quality.* Turnaround time, accuracy, and the ability to call someone you trusted and knew on a first-name basis to deal with problems were favorable points for retaining control of the laboratory. Was this a vote of confidence or a reflection of bad experiences in dealing with national reference labs? Probably some of both. But for the accountants cost was still the key issue.

The Process of Reengineering

Vision/Commitment

First things were first, and that meant a shared vision. Management had to develop a vision that would be significant to everyone and that would keep business and jobs for the future. We needed to share the rationale. We felt that if we didn't undergo reengineering, jobs would be lost. It was important that everyone understand the situation and that we draw from strengths at every level.

The decision to undergo reengineering was made by top management. The reality was that there would be controversy, opposition, and unhappiness, but we all wanted to move forward. We had a forum to discuss the issues for both the hospital and commercial laboratory personnel. The work would be subcontracted if we failed, and fewer employees of the laboratory would remain.

We began by sharing this with all laboratory personnel. These conversations emphasized that our survival was at stake, and this caught their attention. The result was fear and anger directed at management. By this time there were already rumors about the number of positions that would remain. Rumors can be devastating. At Hughes in Tucson, they have a hot line which you can call to discuss any work-related rumor. Although we didn't pursue this option, I felt it was an excellent idea. However, not only is it worthless, but it negatively impacts morale if questions are not answered or answers are untrue. Communication concerning the number of jobs, types of positions, and benefits was critical. I felt the anger as I walked around the lab. If I had lunch with employees at the hospital the most common question I heard was, "Will I have a job?" I also heard this at the commercial lab, although not with the same frequency or level of anxiety. There was a we/they attitude between the two labs that were merging, namely, the commercial and the hospital laboratory personnel. The commercial side continued to grow and prosper because of good management decisions, and a continuing trend to do more in the outpatient area and less with inpatients. The inpatient decisions were controlled by the hospital structure and less flexible. The management was used to a slower decision process and was more reluctant to make changes.

I knew we couldn't just sit back on our laurels, which is often an issue when companies are doing well. (Forty percent of the companies listed in the Fortune 500 in 1980 have now disappeared [3].) A large percentage of the commercial lab personnel would not be affected by the cycling of the positions. This result was perceived as the hospital personnel not being treated fairly. This was partially due to the fact that the staffing at the commercial lab was already fairly efficient and had a good ratio of tests to technicians. Another reason was the uniqueness of positions at the commercial lab. These included couriers, billing, information services, phlebotomy, and processing. The hospital was open 24 hours a day, 7 days a week. But with plans for the core (commercial) laboratory to support the hospital on non-Suprathreshold adaptation tests (STAT; a STAT is required immediately because of the patient's condition) and urgent tests, both sites would be open the same hours. Furthermore, we needed personnel already familiar with the processes and equipment at the core (commercial) laboratory. Standardization of testing and new equipment decisions had to dovetail with equipment depreciation, vendor contracts, and funds available. This would not be done quickly.

The staff needed to know that management was committed to these actions, from the top on down, including our chief executive officer (CEO). Gerry Gilmore, senior vice-president, formerly responsible for only the commercial side, was now in charge of both laboratories. His presence at several forums sent a significant message to personnel, and having one administrative head underlined the reality of the decision to incorporate the two labs and made it clear that it came from top management. Eliminating duplication of top management was a bold move that clearly communicated that we were going to proceed with the reengineering.

A representative group, but predominantly management and pathologists, was formed to develop a shared vision. We first reviewed the system's mission statement: "Caring is our foundation. As leaders, and in collaboration with others, we work with our communities to maintain and improve their health through our comprehensive and integrated health care system. We are committed to providing the best value possible to the customers we serve."

Prior to this, I had participated in forming the system's mission, had heard the message at numerous meetings, and had been part of an effort to make everyone aware of it. During the next year, our mission was made more prominent in all system activities, including posters, newsletters, and the initial prompt of our system E-mail. In addition, progress of change within the system and how it was tied in with the vision was discussed at regularly scheduled meetings of the management, with frequent participation by the system CEO and other top management personnel. However, when I asked lab personnel or fellow physicians about the vision, I was told, "Oh, yeah, caring; something about community." During this time period we had a joint commission on accreditation of hospital inspection, and we tried to get personnel to remember key words like *caring, integrated care,* and *best value.* It is interesting that despite these efforts the vision was not remembered in any detail. We participated in its formation at all levels. A good deal of the effort was wordsmithing, but it did provide direction for the executive leadership. Caring was the value that almost every employee would remember. We developed a short, easily remembered motto: "We get results."

A representative group from both sites began to work on a new mission statement for the laboratory. Over a period of several months, we met outside the laboratory for 2–3 hours. The final results seemed very straightforward. A vision needs to have some meaning to the people formulating it. The initial group was to share stages of development with the rest of the laboratory and encourage, as well as communicate, their input before finalization. This statement was in keeping with the system vision. We knew that there were key words within this statement, including *comprehensive* and *best value.* To me the mission statement was somewhat generic, but it was important that it was a collective effort of both management and employees at multiple levels. The problem remained that even though efforts had been made to invite everyone to participate, only a few did so. The final lab vision statement follows: "As a leader in the medical laboratory field and in partnership with our system, we will provide comprehensive, exceptional, quality service at the best value to the communities and customers we serve."

As time passed, I asked representative personnel in the laboratory if they knew our vision. Generally, I got a shrug of the shoulders, but the key phrases did guide us through some difficult times. We emphasized being a system lab and a member of the system team. Throughout the process we had talked of best value, emphasizing cost and maintaining quality. During this time we had some difficulties and learned a great deal about customers, their expectations, and how to improve our relationship with them. During this time of crisis, quality of service and customer needs were emphasized. I'm not sure how much of the vision statement was originally understood or considered significant. I think that involved personnel were thinking about job security and benefits. However, the emphasis on customers and quality was familiar enough that everyone knew that part of the mission.

LESSON

Even though the mission statement was not remembered, key phrases became almost like a motto.

The Plan

Strategic Priorities

The following are our strategic priorities:

- Name of laboratory—one new name for the two sites
- Reduction in duplication of service
- Development of patient "seamless/hassle-free" laboratory service
- Development of physician "seamless/hassle-free" laboratory service

The system originally had more strategic priorities, which were reduced to customer acquisition, customer retention, and cost reduction. The system strategic priorities were a good fit with ours, serving as a reminder that we should focus on customer issues. We did not list cost reduction, but best value was partially related to cost.

Name. The name of the system was changed during this period. However, because of considerations of changing the name multiple times, with the possibility of a community or regional lab, the lab name was not changed. Finally in May, 6 months after the initiation of the reengineering changes, the name was changed from TMCHE to TMCHE Health Partners Laboratory and ultimately to Health Partners Laboratory of Southern Arizona (HPSA). *TMCHE* stood for "Tucson Medical Center Health Enterprise" and *Health Partners* was the new name for our system. So we were officially HPSA Laboratory, but the signs on vehicles and the buildings read TMCHE, which is still true.

Hassle-free, Seamless Patient and Physician Service. A group composed of pathologists, management, and technical personnel recommended which test would be needed on a STAT basis, regardless of volume. These tests would remain at the hospital. In retrospect, we could have eliminated a good deal of data collection and analysis if we had merely looked at customers' needs. Any test requiring more than an hour to perform was not a STAT test and would detract from the ability of the STAT lab to give a rapid response on other tests requiring a turnaround time of less than 1 hour. This meant educating the clinicians on the reality of potential turnaround time, test by test. We had the clinicians participate in developing this STAT list. (STAT means a test required immediately because of the patient's condition.)

STAT LIST

Chemistry	*Chemistry (continued)*
Acetaminophen/Tylenol	Bilirubin
Acetone	BUN
Alcohol (medical)	Calcium
Ammonia	Carbamazepine (Tegretol)
Amylase	CPK-MB
Apt	*(continued on next page)*

Chemistry
(continued from previous page)

Creatinine

CSF-protein

Drug-of-abuse screen (include tricyclic screen)

Glucose

Iron, total

Lactic acid

Lidocaine

Liver profile (alkaline phosphatase, aspartate aminotransferase, alanine aminotransferase, T&D bili)

Lytes

Mg

Osmolality

Phenobarbital

Phenytoin

Potassium

Pregnancy test (urine/serum screen)

Protein (CSF)

Renal profile (BUN, creat., glucose Cl, CO_2, NaK)

Salicylate

Theophylline

Tricyclic antidepressant screen (drugs of abuse, tricyclics)

Troponin

Uric acid

Blood Bank

ABO/Rh

Direct antiglobulin

Transfusion reaction (work-up)

Type and cross-match (without antibodies)

Head Trauma Coag-Profile

PT, APPT, fibrinogen, D-dimer, CBC

Head Trauma Coag-Profile (continued)

Automatic diff.

Hemo/Coag/Urinalysis

CBC auto

Cell count and diff (CSF)

Coag profile

Complete urinalysis

D-dimer

Fibrinogen

Manual differential

Protamine sulfate time

PT/PTT

SED rate

Thrombin time

Microbiology

Group A strep. screen

Gram stain

HBsAG: Labor and delivery; hemodialysis

Rapid Response List for Tests Ordered as STAT (2-hour turnaround)

Cell count and differential (body fluids)

Haptoglobin

Hyperalimentation panel (glucose, BUN, creatinine, sodium, KCl, CO_2, T-bili, phosphorus, magnesium, calcium, triglycerides, albumin)

Lipase

Lithium

Procainamide/NAPA

Quant. HCG

Quinidine

Sickle cell (for exchange units)

TIBC/iron profile

Valproic acid

Surprisingly, clinicians shortened our original STAT list. We had a rapid-turnaround-time list, which were tests to be completed within 2 hours. These tests were ordered infrequently in the hospital, generally less than 10 per month. Although it made sense economically to do these at the core lab, we ended up bringing some of these back to the hospital. Although they were ordered infrequently, the patient needs were essentially STAT (i.e., a 1-hour or less turnaround time). We also wanted one-call information with a rapid response to any customer concerns (inpatient or outpatient). Previously, section phone numbers were available in the hospital. Thus if you wanted a hematology result you called hematology; for chemistry you called chemistry; and so on. If you weren't sure where to call, you were passed around. The single phone number accessed our client service personnel, who had access to any information, whether it was inpatient or outpatient. In the initial phases there were some disasters, with tests sent to the wrong location, resulting in delays, computer interface problems, and changes in training. Presently, we are completing more than 90% of our STAT tests in the allotted 1 hour. Our goal, which is generally achieved, is 95% of the hospital STAT tests reported in less than 1 hour (from order time to receipt of results).

Duplication. Eliminating duplication of services was a major task involving clinical needs, turnaround time (TAT), equipment, and personnel. Each issue was discussed in detail. Test volumes and cost were evaluated by sections, some of which would later be combined (e.g., hematology and chemistry at the hospital). Each section listed tests and corresponding volumes, and made recommendations on which tests would be needed on a STAT basis in the hospital regardless of volume. This was the key part of the redesign. Only those tests that required STAT would be duplicated. The hospital lab redesign and acquisition of new equipment resulted in a more efficient process. We also discovered cost inefficiencies, such as multiple vendors. In addition, management centralized ordering of supplies, which resulted in fewer vendors, standardization of reagents, and standardization of procedures.

LESSON

Start with customers' needs.
Establish on-site test needs.
Partner with vendors.
Reduce duplication.
Standardize and thereby facilitate cross-training.

Barriers to Success

Barriers fill the gap between current reality and your vision for the future.

BARRIERS

Two computer systems
Severance process not well developed
Fear
We/they attitude between sites
Weak evaluation process
Leadership hierarchy; all leaders not aligned
Distance between staff and customers
First group in the system to undergo reengineering
Short time period to accomplish reengineering

The need for rapid change in health care has created fear. Fear inhibits questioning, participation, and creativity, all of which require risk. Frequently heard comments were: "Will I have a job?" " Will my friends have a job?" The fear of job loss presents a huge barrier. There are no job guarantees, but constantly learning, being creative, and creating value are valuable in any organization. If you do these and you have a team approach and good interpersonal relationships, you will probably have a job. However, if the system fails, then all jobs will disappear, regardless of your qualifications.

If the merger and reorganization were to fail, our lab could not survive, and some wanted failure. They, unrealistically, wanted to return to the previous, more secure situation. A good part of this was related to fear of change. To reduce this anxiety and provide stability, our laboratory leadership promised no more job cuts for at least a year.

Another barrier was the adversarial relationship between management and on-line employees. This was definitely more of an issue at the hospital lab, where key management positions were replaced. To ameliorate this situation we had picnics, a holiday party, and common meetings; these all helped. We also shifted personnel who had worked at one location to the other location, which brought them face to face with the reality of the integration, eliminated many rumors dealing with "they" in the we/they equation, and thereby reduced friction.

With the downsizing and flattening of the organization, some curtailment of promotions was inevitable. Instead of traditional promotions, we would be faced with less middle management and more lower-level responsibility. In the future, power and status that previously came with rank would come with problem-solving ability. The future would mean more coaching and delegating; better feedback, support, and approval; and more training on mentoring and coaching. Moreover, we definitely needed to be better listeners. Coaching in business is not much different from that in sports. We needed to ask, "What are you having problems with?" Then we needed to say, "This is how you kick a football." "This is how you approach problems in business."

Employees want help in learning how to do something, and they want a visible objective. Effective coaching helps all these goals. This restructuring of the roles of our first-level managers was a high priority for us, and it meant additional training, acquiring abilities very different from the traditional role of a laboratory technical manager. Some managers had a hard time relinquishing control. I would listen to team discussions; afterward, in private, managers would list what they were willing to let happen. We had just as many issues with managers not being able to let go of the reins and let the line employees have power as we did with resistance to change by employees. We still have control issues, not just in the lab, but in our entire system. Adapting to change is an ongoing challenge at all levels.

Being first in the system to undergo reengineering, we lacked experienced leadership in the process. Some major processes, such as using the previous evaluations in the selection procedure for rightsizing and individual cycling, posed problems that required creative and rapid solutions. We had set an aggressive goal of 6 months to complete rightsizing, which in our case meant downsizing. In the middle of this turbulence, a prior bid for new business was won, which resulted in a 30% increase in business on the commercial side. Obviously, this affected some of the decisions in downsizing related to the core (commercial) lab.

We had been working on an AHCCCS bid for 6 months. It came through almost at the same moment that we decided to integrate and reengineer. Although testing presented some problems, the primary source of difficulty was the suddenly increased workload for processing. We therefore had to enlarge processing, improve the design, and hire additional personnel for that area.

A major reason to reengineer slowly is that fewer jobs will be cycled, and the rightsizing will occur by attrition. This is an advantage, but with the speed of change in the market, technology, and reimbursement, most organizations cannot afford a long time period.

The Process

Volunteers were accepted for teams, and meetings were assigned leaders. The teams included finance, billing, hospital STAT (rapid turnaround) lab, microbiology, processing, and core lab. This was the beginning of a major effort to get everyone involved. Facilitators from the system helped us, and we encouraged participation and ownership. For example, status reports from the different committees were presented by rotating members from each team rather than by the designated leaders or someone viewed as a manager. This promoted ownership, understanding, and more participation. Making a presentation requires greater understanding, because you must be prepared to answer questions related to any aspect of the presentation.

Empowerment is one of those jargon words we use frequently without stopping to think what it means, which is giving power to someone—power to influence behavior, to make changes as part of a team using collective thought for decision making. The first step in empowerment is to build a foundation of trust based on listening, and then taking action on what has been said. Participants must feel that what they say makes a difference. Action, not words, builds trust. (The consensus decision-making practice we use to build trust and increase levels of accountability is discussed in detail in Chapter 2.)

These self-empowered teams needed to be coached, not directed. We needed to value the employees' input, and they needed to believe that management valued theirs. However, employees needed to understand that although they had considerable freedom, they had to play within the boundaries of the field, which were set by the ability to accomplish our goals and fulfill our vision within the budget, including benefits and wages. Obviously, there were other boundary issues, such as human resource guidelines and the team's abilities and willingness to be accountable. Boundary limitation is an ongoing process.

Teams looked at their processes with a facilitator, emphasizing the redesign of areas and retooling. Strategic priorities for teams were developed. One of the priorities was to let the technical people do the technical work and let lower-level employees do the nontechnical work. The most important priority was to improve the processes and get rid of any step that did not create value.

Letting go of old habits is not easy. We identify and defend positions or processes that we developed and perceived as successful. This change in responsibilities for the positions would result in considerable cost savings because it meant fewer technical positions. For example, previously, technicians were responsible for spinning down the blood, a task now done by someone with less training, who was unable to do the actual testing. We used the technique of asking, "Why?" asking, "Why?" again, and then asking, "What if . . . ?" We did this until we reached an agreeable conclusion. Paradigm shifts resulted in emphasis on speed, flexibility, and innovations. This did not come easy and did not happen overnight.

Mapping the Process

The following had to be decided based on customers' needs before processes could be mapped:

1. Which tests would be done in each location.
2. Which tests could be batched and which needed to be done as they arrived.

Obviously, all tests in the STAT lab would be done as they arrived, making random access equipment (equipment capable of quickly moving high priority tests ahead of others as they arrive) necessary. We then mapped the processes using butcher paper, looking at all handoffs and decision points when the tests could go in several directions. Handoffs were not always efficient. Sometimes neither side of the handoff assumed responsibility, nor did they always look at the previous handoff to see if that was the cause for delay. It became obvious that a more holistic approach, looking at the entire process, was necessary. This meant crossing boundaries of teams we had formed. For example, if turnaround time was the issue, we had to assume some leadership for processes beyond the lab. Turnaround time as perceived by the customer is the time from the doctor's order until the doctor receives the results of the test. Any delays are assumed to be the responsibility of the lab. In the literature, we still see studies of turnaround times that only measure the time in the laboratory. The validity of these traditional studies is questionable. We experienced significant delays before the specimen reached the laboratory and sometimes more extensive delays before the results were read by the physician. We did some random observations to confirm our hypothesis. In the emergency department, we observed multiple tubes of blood being drawn before the patient was seen by the doctor, followed by further delay before the physician's orders. In the computer, the time of the draw was the starting point for the turn around time (TAT) of lab results. Thus we had inaccurate data.

When there is historical ownership of the process by the team members, there is more reluctance to change. Our microbiology team was an example of this. The first time through this process, minimal changes occurred. The workload increased and the questions raised during the initial mapping process were again raised. By this time, there were new technicians with a different viewpoint from those previously involved on a daily basis. With each step in the process, we should ask such questions as, "Why do we need this?" and, "What does it contribute?"

Repeat or duplicate testing was an issue. If the method and process were correct, why would repeat testing be necessary unless there was some inconsistency in the technology? If the data showed no inconsistency, then duplication was eliminated. If lack of precision is a problem, then we should look for new methodology. In retrospect, it is worthwhile to map the process, make changes, and later revisit the process again with outsiders participating. Ask the same questions and you may get different answers. Process change should be ongoing. Once the acceptance of change becomes a way of life, you automatically begin to look at ways to improve on an ongoing basis.

Retool

Standardization of equipment allows greater flexibility of cross-training for different locations and more cost-effective purchasing of large volumes of reagent. Standardization also supported workstation consideration. Flexibility meant random access or batch mode, open channels for future testing, and freedom to use more than one manufacturer's reagent. As far as reliability went, we were unwilling to be the first to try a new piece of equipment unless we were to be a beta-testing site and get some form of reimbursement for our time. We didn't have time to be working out the kinks with a new piece of equipment. With this in mind, we developed a matrix for equipment selection.

A matrix equipment acquisition should be developed by every institute according to their needs. Following are some suggested areas covered:

Reagents: Number of tests per container, reagent cost, reagent volumes, storage, stability, time to prepare

Sampling: Random access, bar codes, sample size, test per hour

Computer: Type of data storage, used independently, two-way compatibility, interface, machine-generated labels, bar code reader

Optical system: Types of cuvets, number of photometer systems, light source, life of light source

Calibration: Time required, frequency, frequency of controls, cost of controls

Installation: Water, electrical, drain

Maintenance: Time required, availability of outside maintenance

Miscellaneous: Hotline and/or telephone modem for troubleshooting

Future capabilities

Reputation of company

Comments from users

Evaluations and Downsizing

Before the process of evaluations we had a dollar reduction figure as a goal. It became evident very quickly that we could not reach this goal without reduction in full-time equivalents. During the process reviews, the participants knew that there would be fewer personnel with a greater workload, but, it was hoped, with greater efficiency. By combining chemistry, urinalysis, and hematology, and by redesigning the space, we eliminated sample handling and a number of walking steps. Eventually, we reduced personnel by 20%. We cut 40 full-time equivalents (FTEs) while maintaining necessary skills. The timetable did not allow us to do this by attrition.

Previous evaluations had been based on performance but they were not well done. Initially, our human resources people had said that we would do the reengineering with downsizing based on seniority, but when we looked at other institutions that had already gone through this process, we learned that it was best done by looking at individual performance. The previous evaluations were almost worthless. Some personnel we knew had performed poorly but had been rated as exceeding standards. In the past, raises were based on a rating of "exceeds standards," and most received that rating. Evaluations were done by a supervisor with little other input, and the avoidance of confrontation was a priority.

A group of people in management sought input from employees and directly participated in evaluating every person employed by the lab. This group included three people from outside the lab who shared available performance evaluations and whose job was to maintain some consistency in the decision process. This was an emotionally difficult period. The three independent observers who participated gave good feedback on the content of the discussion and helped focus the group. It was amazing that our scores matched on more than 90% of the people. We placed them in one of three categories: *limited capacity, meets standards,* or *exceeds standards.* Technical knowledge and ability were high priorities, but interpersonal skills and being a team player were equally important. A good performer who was not a team player could create internal sabotage and be a disaster for the outcome of the reengineering. Those in the limited command group were offered a severance package or early retirement, depending on age, or they could take 45 days (this is called the cycle time) to redeploy to another job within the system. After this we began to do an annual 360-degree evaluation, which included input from peers who worked with the employees or were in a position to observe them.

Denial to Acceptance. The downsizing resulted in a grieving process. According to Kubler-Ross, the first stage in any grieving process is denial. When reduction became a reality, we were in the stage of active resistance or anger. During this stage the technical training occurred in the STAT lab for the added individual responsibility. Because of this we needed to have cycled personnel available to cover shifts. Morale was at an all-time low. Employees felt that management was unfair to those who were leaving, and those who stayed were concerned that they might be next, and probably felt guilty that they were still employed. It took about 3 months to get into the "emergent" stage, where personnel recognized that the changes were not that bad. It took approximately 1 year to reach the experimenting stage, where personnel start to truly move on and have a sense of direction (4).

Cycling. Before downsizing, review the following:

In-source work previously sent out
Consider the potential for cutting the workweek across the board
Develop new product lines
Market more aggressively

Employees who were part of the laboratory downsizing were given several options. They could stay in the system if they successfully redeployed to another job, in which case they would receive no severance pay. They could leave the system, receiving severance pay and benefits related to age and number of years worked in the system. If they were reemployed in the system, they could apply for a job, be interviewed first, and have the job offer or refusal immediately. This did not work well for managers because they limited themselves to seeing one candidate. Because of this, many saw hiring those in cycle as a disadvantage.

We obtained outside counseling for jobs, but no specific training was offered. There was financial support for those going back to school. There was help with resume composition, interview skills, and information services for jobs available in our area or in other parts of the country. Because we outsourced the reemployment, we got very little feedback. In retrospect, we should have spent more time doing follow-up to learn more about opportunities for improvement of this important process. Since then, redeployment training has become an internal operation of the system.

Several of the cycled middle managers returned to the bench, applying for new positions that eventually became available. This was an emotional time. We realized that when someone lost his or her job, it frequently meant leaving a job that supported a family. I wish there was an easier way to do this. Our system employed 5,000 people in a variety of positions, but most who were cycled had special laboratory skills and wanted to continue working in laboratory medicine. A few were close to retirement and did not return to work. Several went to other fields successfully, including computer sales and tax accounting. Some found work in other laboratories in the city. It is very difficult to accept that you were released as a result of peer performance comparison. Seniority doesn't work as well as a selective process for the organization, but it is unquestionably easier on the individual's ego. Nonetheless, when you look at your objectives, you must choose performance if you want a highly motivated and successful team.

In-house family services offered free counseling. Most of the explanations of benefits were done individually, which was felt to be more sensitive. In retrospect, doing this in large groups would have resulted in additional questions, including issues that individuals may not have thought of but that were equally important. Looking back, we felt that initiating more per diem positions from the phase of inception would have allowed us more flexibility, and we would have been in a position to cycle fewer personnel.

Morale would have been stronger and the process would have moved more rapidly and been more positive if those in cycle could have left immediately after they were informed. I am not sure if there was any way to do this while satisfying training needs. Once the individuals in cycle left, there was a positive quantum leap in morale. One option would be to give those who are cycled out the option of staying and working for a certain time or leaving immediately. Those who stayed would be paid a bonus if they performed to expectation, which would include being supportive of the reengineering and system goals. This has been tried at other institutions and has worked well.

Communication/Changing Goals

Sharing information successfully is difficult, especially when many are in denial. We used forums, posted minutes, and asked involved personnel from the initial group section meetings to take the information back to their sections for discussion. We needed input so that the personnel would be part of the process.

Successful change requires acceptance and participation. To accept change you must feel that it is going to make things better. Generally, you adapt by changing things slightly so that they are unique for you. It takes time and effective communication to go from observer, to occasional player, to active participant. Top management needed to learn to communicate better, to be more flexible, and to step back and let others take control within established guidelines. They also knew that goals would change, as trigger events occur that make you reconsider your strategy. For example, one of the goals in microbiology was to have no incoming phone calls. But after negative input from some key clinicians, we realized that the infectious disease physicians and a few pulmonary specialists wanted results before they were available in the computer, or available to our client service representatives handling the phone inquiries. The decision was made to allow a limited number of infectious disease personnel and pulmonary staff to use the direct number to microbiology. Nevertheless, we eliminated a full-time technical position from microbiology because of significant reduction of incoming phone calls. In addition, we realized that many results were unavailable, such as early-morning orders for cultures taken the day before. It turned out that many hospital cultures ordered early in the day were not received in the laboratory until late in the evening. We began a campaign to receive these cultures earlier, thus having the results available to the physicians when they made rounds. In addition, we encouraged the doctors to check the nursing unit monitors for more up-to-date results. We were not a paperless system, and the number of doctors who used the hospital information system was limited. But if it paid dividends by not having to call the lab, perhaps this would be a first step in the process of having the doctors use the computer. Note that the most important part of the process was fine-tuning the timely receipt of specimens from the nursing units.

Communication must be frequent, allow input, and be received from those considered leaders. For this to happen, leaders must be visible and available as much as possible. If there is no effective communication, then rumors will fill the vacuum, with devastating results. Communicate data on progress toward specific goals. There remains a fine balance between input, decision making, and achievement of goals. Input and communication are great, but decisions have to result in achievement of goals. Failure remains the responsibility of top leadership.

Informing Our Customers. If you communicate effectively and eliminate surprise regarding service, you will have greater customer satisfaction in difficult times. Hoping to develop a closer relationship, we assigned pathologists and management to nursing units. We made ourselves more visible in the nursing units by making rounds with some frequency. We established nurse/unit clerk bimonthly meetings, resulting not only in constructive criticism, but some positive feedback. This was attended by nurses, unit clerks, pathologists, medical technologists, and management. People began to know one another on a first-name basis, helping build much-needed relationships. In the initial phase, there were disasters in turnaround times because of specimens misplaced, delayed, or wrong test order. It was not a smooth transition.

We initiated a problem log phone number. We asked those involved to call a specific number, relay the information, and wait for someone to get back to them. This information was typed and distributed to key personnel Monday through Friday. The follow-up was formally typed and recorded, allowing us to see the problem resolution and giving the lab some idea of the frequency of the problems. Even this did not go smoothly. We eventually assigned a specific person to this task. This individual had computer skills to track problems and worked closely with managers and pathologists to improve the processes. In addition, this troubleshooter made rounds in the units on a regular basis, sometimes accompanied by technicians, laboratory information personnel, or pathologists. The individual had responsibility for publishing a turnaround time on the most frequent chemistry profile and urinalysis for the emergency department, as well as partial thromboplastin times for the critical care areas. This was done every month and represented the turnaround time for the previous week. We shared this information with our staff and the staff of those units. Communications of the progressive improvement of turnaround time in the hospital improved the lab's image.

Physician Communication. The 100 top physician admitters to the hospital were divided up among the pathologists and were visited in their offices. These physicians were given the opportunity to discuss how they felt about the reengineering and to know what to expect. It is often said that if you know what is coming, you are more willing to accept an issue than if you have no knowledge of it. We didn't want people to be surprised. In talking to and/or visiting other laboratories that had gone through reengineering, one of the things consistently stressed was the need to communicate well with the physicians. We went to every medical meeting for an entire month and put reengineering on the agenda for discussion. We went with a potential list of STAT tests that would stay in the hospital and those that would be sent to the core lab, our off-site facility. We knew that it was important that the physicians participate in a discussion of their needs, focusing on tests that would be done on-site with a 1-hour turnaround time.

The discussion with the physicians emphasized why we were undergoing reengineering and integration, and the positive aspects for them. What would be the advantages? These included more frequent testing of some of the esoteric procedures and ability to incorporate outpatient with inpatient results. Thus one phone call would give them the results they needed. Prior to this, they would call the outpatient lab and be irritated when they could not get the result, remaining unaware that this source did not have the results from the hospital testing. Access to preadmission testing of patients for hospitalization was facilitated, resulting in less duplication and more efficient patient care. By creating a specific area for STATs and taking all routine testing out of the hospital, we promised that STAT testing would turn around faster. Although this was not the case initially, within 6 months we had achieved a 1-hour TAT on 96% of the emergency department testing. Publishing this information diluted complaints about the uncommon variations that are always brought up as though the anecdotal experience represented the most frequent occurrence. The physicians stressed the need for retention of service and accuracy, and we stressed the same in the data we provided for them. It is important to make frequent visits and ask, "How are we doing?" A thank you for all criticisms—because they present an opportunity for improvement—is equally important.

Guidelines for Talking to Physicians Regarding Lab Integration
1. Why are we doing this?
   a. Increase the efficiency of the service, making it more cost-effective.
   b. Look at ways to cut costs to third party payers including Partners, Medicare, etc.
   c. Cut duplication where it does not affect patient care.
   d. Provide continuity between the inpatient and outpatient labs.
   e. Improve STAT turnaround time.
   Note: The goal is to cut costs in the first year by $800,000.
2. The advantages:
   a. True STATs may actually turn around faster.
   b. Central client services (i.e., one phone call for either outpatient or inpatient after November) will result.
   c. Hospital results can be pulled up through Physician Link and eventually TMCHE (outpatient) results can be obtained through this same link.
   d. More tests can be done locally.
   e. On some of the more esoteric tests because of the combined volume, there will be more frequent testing.
   f. This will position us for future health maintenance organization bids to keep the work local.
3. What do we need from them?
   a. There may be some issues in the first couple of weeks. Please do not increase the number of STAT orders.
   b. Understanding and patience.
   c. Communication of issues so that they can be resolved.
   d. If there is a problem, please call one of the pathologists and talk to them about the issues. It is hoped that will help resolve the issue.

Possible Objections from the Doctors
How can we have true STAT service when it is out of the hospital?

Response: The STAT list was developed with the help of the Emergency Room physicians and should satisfy any immediate needs that the patient will have. Are there additional changes they would like to suggest?

I'm going to order everything STAT.

Response: We are way above the national average of 35%, which includes the Emergency Room. We can't cut costs with this attitude.

The nurses' comment on STATs was, "We need to educate the docs."

Doctors' objections: "I want it to stay the way it is."

Health care reform: Everything is changing, including pressures on the laboratory to reduce costs without reducing significant service. There was actually a group from the hospital that met to look at using a national lab and keep only STAT lab services in the hospital.

Cost Objection

I want a peripheral lab.

Response: An additional lab in the emergency department or the critical care areas would necessitate expensive equipment and FTEs that are not available and would drive up the costs significantly. We have to first increase the efficiency of use of a pneumatic tube that went directly to the lab. If it does not positively affect the outcome, it is not cost-effective. We are doing as much point-of-care testing as any hospital in the country.

I'm going to order everything on the 3:00 A.M. run so that I can have it on the chart when I make rounds.

Response: The original implications of the 3:00 A.M. run were that it was for the intensive care area. It has now been expanded to the entire hospital. It certainly should not be used for routines or for rehabilitation patients unless *absolutely* necessary. For the 3:00 A.M. run, the vast majority will be on the chart by 6:00 A.M., certainly those tests on the STAT list.

We did not spend enough effort organizing and planning training, which resulted in insufficient training. We were not unique in this regard. Others who were also undergoing reengineering echoed the theme over and over again. This deficiency was overcome, but with difficulty, primarily because of the sudden overload of additional work for which we were unprepared.

No amount of planning will eliminate every problem. Take a course of action that allows you to deal with unanticipated issues and smooth out the processes. There was enough concern about accuracy and caring for the outcomes related to patients that superlative effort by all personnel was seen during this time. We needed to balance the training and move forward from the drawing board fairly quickly to prevent apathy.

Additional Barriers

Cross-training on Computers and Equipment. We tried not to rehire in areas of attrition. We were very busy and it was difficult to find time for training. Many people were still angry and not fully cooperative. We had two different computer software systems—one for the hospital and another for the commercial lab—connected with an interface. In retrospect this was unwise, but at the time we thought we could not afford to change it. Buying an additional system and bringing up new software would also create problems. Given our budget, we felt we didn't have a choice. If we had gone to one computer, we would have had more flexibility in rotating personnel between the hospital lab and the core lab. Many of the service issues were related to problems of interfacing the computers. For example, the interface program did not initially accept add-on orders. This created a real problem because the processing personnel of the hospital did not know that these orders were not being received at the core lab. Once discovered, that correction was made quickly.

In retrospect, the following should have occurred:

1. Provide more planned time for training.
2. Give a specific schedule for individual training in the technical areas.
3. Everyone to redo lab orientation including our new mission statement.
4. Encourage input concerning changes from personnel who have worked elsewhere.
5. Involve key personnel who enjoyed teaching.
6. Make training continuous.

Billing. Before the reengineering, the hospital accounting department was responsible for billing institutions on campus. This included a psychiatric center and an orthopedic institute. The commercial side had billing responsibility for outpatients (excluding those that went through the hospital). There were different prices for the hospital and commercial lab institutions. This policy was eliminated, and all referring commercial institutions were billed through the outpatient billing department with increased efficiency.

Rewards. Throughout the processes, celebrating successes was a key issue that we could have improved on. Our celebrations included the IZAP program, in which the more IZAP dollars you had, the more valuable the reward was. For example, one potential purchase with multiple IZAP (a program in which managers or fellow employees would give fake dollars called IZAP to any employee they caught doing something positive) dollars was a week-end at a local resort. If an effort was superlative, such as an emergency that required doing the work of two people and working overtime with almost no breaks, you could receive more than one IZAP dollar. Unfortunately, we did not use this program as often as we should have. We also had a suggestion program that rewarded people in the same manner or with a $25 gift certificate. There were no limits to the number of suggestions one individual could make in a week, month, quarter, or year. Suggestions had to meet one or more of the following criteria: improve customer service, improve safety, improve productivity, or reduce costs. Suggestions were to be as specific as possible. If information was insufficient, the manager responsible for that area was asked for clarification and/or more data. Self-directed work teams within the laboratory were encouraged to keep track of the ideas they implemented within their work unit and to submit them for review and payment.

Outcome

The merger and reengineering process between the hospital and the core lab was a success. Changes continue, and in an Ernst & Young survey, our cost per test was the lowest of 15 hospitals and competitive with national reference laboratories. We have also merged with another lab (owned by an 80-physician group), which eliminated duplication of testing and equipment and reduced the number of required personnel. This reduction was achieved by attrition rather than layoffs. We are committed to standardization of equipment and testing for the three merged labs. We have ended up saving almost double our initial goal. Processes continue to be revamped. The hospital problem log, originally up to two pages per day, now averages only a few instances per week. But in health care, the goal is zero defects.

LESSONS LEARNED

These are some of the lessons we learned:

1. Have specific goals that can be appreciated and achieved, separate from your mission/vision.
2. Establish a dialogue with managed care, including how you can help each other.
3. Remember that best value means accuracy, service, and costs. Accuracy and service are assumed.
4. Discuss changes personally with key physicians.
5. Try to avoid surprises.
6. Communicate strategic priorities to all employees.
7. Communicate and listen.
8. Use multiple communication forums (small groups, posters, E-mail, and so on).
9. Stress communication between the supervisor and the on-line employees.
10. Locate testing related to customers' needs.
11. Deal with rumors on a timely basis; consider a rumor hot line.
12. Processes should be revisited on an ongoing basis.
13. Let the technicians do the technical work.
14. Have outsiders participate in any process discussion.
15. Formalize ongoing training related to specific needs.
16. If possible, once informed of status, remove cycled employees from the job.
17. After downsizing, offer some job security.
18. Develop and use performance evaluation indicators.
19. Move personnel between locations during mergers.
20. Cycle based on performance not seniority.
21. With regard to hiring practices, offer some advantage for cycled employees but do not structure to the disadvantage of those hiring.

SUMMARY

With the continuous change in health care, more and more organizations need to make a quantum leap in performance to survive. Reengineering represents a radical change related to process refinement, resulting in improvement. Reengineering requires careful planning boldly embarked on and reasonably balanced with action. Lessons learned from this experience are many. We must learn from our failures, seeing them as opportunities for improvement. Reengineering is an ongoing process and, like life, is a journey. Change is our traveling companion.

REFERENCES

1. Hammer M, Stanton SA: *Re-engineering revolution handbook*, vol. 3. New York: Harper Business, 1995, p. 315.
2. Bellewether Scenario, Sczchs Group: Benchmarking, data rules. *Hospital & Health Network Magazine* 1997:32.
3. Imparato N, Harari O: *Jumping the curve*. San Francisco: Jossey-Bass, 1984, p. 82.
4. Kubler-Ross E: *Questions and answers on death and dying*. New York: Macmillan, 1974, p. 16.

2

Leadership Imperatives

Joni S. Condit

Health care is in various stages of transformation across the United States because of marketplace demands to reduce the cost of care while simultaneously increasing access to care. This transformation began first in California, Arizona, Massachusetts, and Minnesota. Managed care has been the vehicle for the transformation, usually in the form of a fixed amount of dollars for the care of a specified population. Managing care for a fixed amount of money has required a transformation in health care leaders. This chapter chronicles the ongoing effort of one health care organization to meet these marketplace challenges and the crucial changes that have resulted.

CENTERING ON WHAT IS VALUED

It was a hot July day in the Tucson desert, not the time of year normally selected by local companies to work on corporate goals. Our new hospital administrator had gathered some 100 people together to begin redesigning the delivery of care in our hospital, an institution that had survived and prospered for more than 50 years. Physicians, nurses, ancillary clinical leaders, business managers, board members, staff, and facilitators sat in two large concentric circles in a large conference room.

To the few in the room who realized it, this was a community where managed care had come to dominate more than 65% of the market by 1995. Intense competition was causing revenues to decline rapidly. The administrator knew what many in the room did not yet accept or understand: major changes in the delivery of health care from this hospital organization would have to be implemented rapidly if it was to survive. He knew that the 100 present would have to pull together to set their course of action, focusing on a limited number of critical improvements, convincing others to develop a better way of working with one another in caring for patients.

"Pick a partner near you. Go outside or somewhere away from the rest of the group and tell your partner a story, a personal story that represents why you were drawn to work in health care. Visualize and describe that scene in detail." After the group returned to the room, the facilitator asked everyone to sit down, be very quiet, and close their eyes. Soft, beautiful music played during a quiet meditation period, which was followed by the facilitator's soothing voice. The facilitator explained that the session would allow people to speak up when they wanted, without pressure, and to share the story that had just been shared with their partner.

At first the group was silent; then one person quietly came forth with her story. This manager, Jan, had fiercely represented a group of elderly patients suffering from chronic problems, who regularly used the hospital swimming pool to fight their crippling diseases. In the face of a cost reduction plan to eliminate the pool, she championed their cause, citing the pool's social and medical necessity. Jan spoke of the thank you card she unexpectedly received from these individuals for her efforts, and how much this meant to her.

Then came the story from the director of surgery, who explained that early in her career she had cared for a frightened young Catholic woman, who had made the difficult decision to have an abortion. The nurse told the room with a choked voice how she, also a Catholic, had prayed with the woman and had held her hand as the woman went to the operating room. The nurse said that she knew she had made a difference in that patient's life by supporting her in a crisis.

The next story was of an elderly married couple who had both been critically injured in a car accident but were at two different hospitals. The nurses from our hospital realized that the husband and wife were not progressing as well as they might have if they had been together. The nurses had unsuccessfully lobbied the couple's health plan and the other hospital's management to share in expenses for an ambulance to bring the husband to see his wife. The other hospital refused to help out financially. Finally, with the cooperation of our hospital's administration, our nurses hired the ambulance and brought the husband to see his wife. Both husband and wife had nearly given up hope, thinking that the other was dying. Upon being reunited, the couple began to improve dramatically. Shortly after, both were released to go home.

Many stories were told. At one point, the hospital administrator began to tell his story. It was a very recent story of visiting his dying father in Bogotá, Colombia, where the administrator had been born. In grief, he was reunited with his brothers and sisters. One night after his father had died, the administrator had a dream about a bear. It was a fierce bear and the survival of the man depended upon his facing the bear. The bear represented his own fear; the fear of losing his father. There was great emotion in the voice of the administrator. It was an intensely personal and gripping moment, shared with 100 people, many of whom were relative strangers.

The effect of the stories was powerful. They moved many to tears. Not one story had to do with efficiency or making money. In two short hours, the values of 50 years were shared in the storytelling. Several facilitators captured the key points of the stories on flip charts quietly off to the side. These values were the foundation of the organization, the essence of what was sacred and must be preserved no matter what else came to be. The stories underscored why people dedicate their lives to caring for the ill. They told of sharing some of the most private and important moments of families, of life's greatest transitions—birth, death, illnesses, and recovery. It was clear by the end of this session what our long-term purpose as an organization had been. It was also clear that our mission would continue to be the commitment to caring for patients and their loved ones.

Once our group had centered on the values that were honored by the institution, groups of eight to 10 individuals were asked to focus on current reality. Having agreed on what we valued, it was relatively easy to identify those processes that clearly needed repair. Bonded by the earlier events of the day, the groups were able to have intimate dialogues about the issues that were plaguing the hospital and interfering with the smooth care of patients and their families. The 100-member group reconvened after lunch to rank the order of the top four processes most in need of redesign. In that afternoon, the entire group committed to a new method of work, to the major changes required to meet our commitments to patient care. At the end of the day, everyone was asked to stand to signify their support of changing the entire hospital organization and to support the principles of patient-focused care. The attendees left the room, unanimous in support of the changes required. Two years later, the commitments made that day were summarized in writing to be given to patients upon their admission to our hospital. The statement goes as follows:

Tucson Medical Center

Caring Is Our Foundation

Our Commitment to You (the Patient):

We recognize that any visit to the hospital may be a time of stress and concern for you, your family, and friends. The staff of Tucson Medical Center will honor the trust you and your doctor have placed in us by applying our professional ethics, knowledge, and skills to best serve your physical, emotional, and spiritual needs.

- In all aspects of your care, we will keep you well informed and involved in the decision-making. Your preferences and needs will be respected. Information you share with us will be held in confidence.
- To provide you with the finest care, we will strive to establish an individualized and attentive relationship with you and those important to you. Our staff will attend to your needs through appropriate and sensitive responses.
- We will communicate effectively with each other to coordinate your care and treatments.
- We will strive to deliver as much of your care as possible at the bedside.
- We will provide a health care team with the best knowledge, skills, and technology to benefit your health and well-being.
- If you feel we have not lived up to this commitment, please let any member of our health care team know.

The Staff of Tucson Medical Center

The participants left the July retreat understanding clearly what they collectively valued and what motivated them to come to work each day. They were focused on four processes that required complete support of the organization to repair and change. The members of the group knew that their work on these processes would be in the context of what would be best for the patient. The way to do this remained in question.

THE ROLE OF LEADERS

Most employees want to do the right thing—to come to work each day, dedicated to giving their best and doing something worthwhile. Many cannot articulate the higher purpose or the long-term mission toward which they want to strive. Leaders play a critical role in articulating a compelling, altruistic reason for the hard work and sacrifice that each employee will face. Leaders must be able to describe why change is needed before employees will endorse it. The ability of an organization to mobilize its efforts to survive and to succeed depends on its leaders' ability to convey the story so that all employees understand the need to make a commitment and take appropriate action.

Soon after the retreat, the administrator reconvened the entire group but focused this time on the middle management team. He emphasized that success this year would require significant improvement in four of the core processes of the hospital. To achieve this, managers would have to demonstrate key accountabilities. Our administrator outlined the following accountability for middle management:

Management Accountability

Leadership

You should be able to:

- Describe to your staff the role of management in their mission to care for the patients.
- Articulate what our health care system and hospital vision is and how to achieve it.

- Articulate the *essential* aim of each staff team.
- Define, prioritize, and resolve both internal and external customer concerns.
- *Create* a sense of momentum.
- Accept accountability for the daily operating discipline, the processes they serve, and the human behaviors that make them work.
- Deal with your staff in a straightforward and direct manner and demonstrate to staff that you are available and involved.
- Actively pursue continuous education and serve as a role model in all that you do and say.
- Demonstrate to staff that they are supported when working to do the right things in the right way.
- Build effective relationships to help staff get their work accomplished.

Quality

You and your line staff should be able to:

- Understand the basic principles of Continuous Quality Improvement and *why* this is the key to your success.
- Use flowcharts to define all key internal and external processes.
- Define and measure performance toward meeting key customer requirements for cycle time, cost, and service quality using statistical process control tools such as histograms, run charts, control charts, etc.
- Describe through flowcharts hospital/health care system processes that the area supports.
- Establish a value point that your staff will optimize.
- Work productively with other hospital teams.

Human Relations

You and your staff should understand:

- How they are compensated.
- How they can address human resource issues.
- How they are disciplined and why.
- Why the staff reduction policy exists.
- What the *staff* reduction policy is and what protections are built in for employees and how the policy could be applied.
- How their personal behavior and their team behavior determines their success, and ultimately the organization's.
- That guidelines/policies are applied fairly and evenly throughout our hospital.
- How to communicate within the organization.
- How to organize as teams to have productive dialogue and inquiry.
- That management will help correct organization/department behaviors that demonstrate disrespect to the staff.
- That staff are important and that management works to support them.

Resource Utilization

You and your staff should be able to:

- Understand a balance sheet and profit and loss statement: How they are the ultimate indicator of financial strength.
- Understand *budgets* of all processes in which they serve.
  What value the process adds.
  How to measure the performance of the process.
  Be aware of established benchmarks in industry to compare what gaps exist between optimal performance and the current system.
  Be able to use statistical process control (SPC) to monitor performance.
  Be able to make resource allocation decisions.
- Be knowledgeable about what business they are in and how they are reimbursed.
- Understand what response management *will* likely have to changing market conditions.
- Understand how the hospital and your work unit has *balanced* the utilization of resources.

The accountabilities that our hospital administrator identified for middle managers were broader and more encompassing than most had been asked to assume in the past. Demonstration of these accountabilities was critical if our organization was to make the transition to peak performance in a managed-care environment. In health care today, middle managers must be able to perform in a number of roles: leaders of their own departments, redesign pacesetters, team members in some projects, team leaders in others; they must be able to focus one hour on strategy and the next on clinical or technical issues, to perform as a financial analyst, and to act as a coach. The traditional lines between departments have blurred, as have the differences between employees and managers. More and more of the work and decision-making occurs in teams. Some teams are temporary, some are ongoing, and some are created for long-term projects. All these changes enhance the participation and accountability of every employee for the fate of the organization.

RESTRUCTURING TO TRANSFER ACCOUNTABILITY TO STAFF

Like most health care institutions, ours was organized by a traditional command-and-control structure, one that had been very paternalistic toward middle management and line staff. The emphasis on cost containment and related downsizing of middle management made the tradition of unilateral centralized control impractical. Senior leaders in this situation found themselves inundated with minor and major operational decisions and little time for strategic planning. The reductions of middle management required senior leaders to eliminate requirements for approval of every decision. In a flattened organization, a successful manager must work collaboratively, share control and decision-making. For operations to flow smoothly, an effective leader must learn to advocate, coach, and influence, so that many decisions are made by the staff closest to the customer.

A shift in accountability to middle managers and to staff is essential to improving service to the customer. The learning process for staff requires their managers to be effective role models. In a recent example, our physical therapy manager was paged by her staff because of a dilemma created by the high winter volume of inpatients. She called from another patient area to learn that a patient's discharge would be delayed by a day because the hospital was out of crutches, which this patient required. The manager and the therapists quickly decided to call a local durable medical equipment store. One of the therapists drove the several blocks to obtain the crutches in time for the patient to be discharged as planned.

A market-driven organization, in contrast to the traditional command-and-control company, is fast-paced and much less hierarchical. Skills, competencies, and influence are more highly valued than position or title. In our organization, an example of an individual with influential power is the leader of the Continuous Quality Improvement Group. The leader, Kathy, began facilitating teams and teaching quality improvement skills. She is an excellent communicator who demonstrates a deep understanding of the institution and the managed-care market. Although she has relatively little statutory power, her influence is evident. She is included in nearly every strategic planning session and consulted by any team seeking to make significant quality improvements.

Making the transition from a command-and-control, hierarchical structure to one that is flatter, responsive, and more customer focused is not easy. After the energizing retreat, the hospital administrator knew that he had to do something to break the traditional chains of power. The implementation of "patient-focused" care as the model in our hospital, in conjunction with the four significant organization-wide process improvement initiatives, required cross-functional teams. The departmental management boundaries had to be crossed if core processes were to improve.

The administrator developed five teams to "rebalance" the company. The members of these teams, recommended by their peers, were created to represent 25% staff, 25% management, and 50% physicians. Because of patient appointment schedules and dissatisfaction with payer reimbursements, physician participation has been difficult to maintain, with the exception of the Human Resources Team. The physicians involved in this group have been very committed to improving employee morale.

The Human Relations Balancing Team, led by the health system medical director, serves as the interface between the hospital's staff and the Human Resources Department. The Leadership Balancing Team was founded to decide what the new structure and leadership of the organization should be. The Human Resources Team gathered to develop the necessary tools for middle managers and staff to manage the resources of the organization. The System Integration Balancing Team's role was to aid in identifying and eliminating barriers to integrating the hospital with other divisions of the organization and with the community. It also undertook a project to develop a model for identifying, benchmarking, and measuring customer satisfaction with the core processes of the hospital, so that improvements could be made and collaboration with outside organizations could be facilitated. Finally, the Continuous Quality Improvement Team was created as the primary balancing team and was given trusteeship for major cross-functional quality improvements in the organization.

Despite the balancing teams, it became clear that the lack of agreement among senior leaders about the appropriate structure of the organization was challenging the congruity and unity of the organization. This organization was comprised of a tertiary-care hospital with a busy trauma/emergency department, a psychiatric hospital, a children's rehabilitation clinic, a commercial laboratory that served the system and the community, an orthopedic complex, an oncology complex, a corporate division, 120 employed physicians, and part ownership in a statewide managed-care corporation. The flattened organization was still sluggish because some middle managers were stymied, waiting for senior management to agree on structure, focus, and plans for the future.

COMMITMENTS TO INTERNAL CUSTOMERS TO FOSTER CHANGE

In the hospital, the largest part of the organization, it was increasingly clear that we needed key organizing principles to foster internal integration to reach our goals.

The Human Relations Balancing Team began to address some of this need by focusing on the underlying values of the organization. Studying a number of organizations and comparing them with our own, the group developed the following value statements:

Caring: Supporting mutual physical, emotional, and spiritual needs of staff members, and working towards the best outcomes in all we do. Exhibiting compassion, honesty, attention, nurturing, and kindness.

Respect: Honoring the uniqueness of each other; offering understanding, equality, integrity, and commitment.

Service: Giving our best for our communities: demonstrating encouragement, sharing, unselfishness, forgiveness, leadership, humility, and joy in our work.

Personal accountability: Contributing personal and professional talents, committing to appropriate and financially sound actions; speaking the truth with sensitivity.

Learning: Building individual, team, and organizational wisdom and skills, admitting and learning from mistakes; encouraging openness, questioning, dialogue, risk-taking, creativity, and teaching.

Teamwork: Working in unit: fostering synergy and collaboration; sharing knowledge, responsibility, and credit.

These six basic values were shared with middle management and staff for reflection and revision. Once adopted, the Human Relations Balancing Team decided that if identifying these values was to be of any use, they should be the basis of every key decision made by anyone in the organization. The group developed a small yellow card called the Value-Based Decision Card. On one side were printed the six values and their definitions. On the other side were the questions that team members should ask themselves as they made decisions or evaluated if they had conducted themselves in a manner consistent with our organizational values.

The questions are as follows:

• Am I certain that the decision reached is based on accurate information?
• Have I thought through how this decision will affect others?
• Do I understand the financial impact of this decision?
• Did I support the common good over my bias and opinions?
• Do I understand how this decision supports our mission?
• Do I agree with this decision? If not, will I support it?
• Was I respectful and respected during the decision-making process?

These values were important, but more was needed than organizing principles. With a recent decision to forego a merger with another regional health care organization, and the seeming "disintegration" with our own health plans, there was doubt about the integrity of the organization's purpose. It had been three years since the organization had stated its mission and constructed its three-year vision. Much had changed in that time.

The hospital administrator began a dialogue with his managers about the organization's purpose and asked whether they thought that senior leaders of the larger health care organization were committed fully to this purpose. The group, slow to respond and tentative, began over several weeks to discuss the dysfunctions of the organization, particularly in key support areas. The long-term mission of caring for people through some of life's greatest and most difficult transitions was still credible and worthwhile to the managers, but some suspected that some of their senior leaders had lost their commitment and focus. Many commented about failure to "walk the talk." Clinical leaders identified the specific examples of where support systems had broken down, handoffs that did not occur properly, and work that consequently had to be done again. Action plans were generated with specific time tables and accountabilities. These were forwarded to the senior executives of these support areas.

Specific improvements followed, beginning with the need to address below-market compensation rates for certain key positions. Computers were provided where they were especially needed. A "summer of learning" training plan was developed to ensure that new employees would be fully trained and ready for a busy fall.

COMMITMENT TO LEARNING

The health delivery system is a product of the way its employees think and interact. The primary leverage therefore lies not in its policies, budgets, or organizational charts, but in its human resources and the culture of the organization. To develop capacities to change and improve these patterns of thinking and interaction, the organization must commit to learning.

Much has been written describing the essence of good leadership. The truth is that good leadership skills are formed early. Some, such as analytical skills, can be learned, but communication skills are difficult to acquire for those who lack the natural art. Learned leadership requires an environment that, in health care, extends from the spiritual to the physical. This means achieving personal mastery in areas of reflection, conversation, and self-awareness. Open dialogue with peers and good mentors support this development. From the physical aspect, there must be available resources, tools, and technologies that allow better communication, practice fields, and forums for learning. Leaders must move from the position of telling to creating opportunities for employees to experience.

Among the most difficult times that a leader may face are when great change is required and its outcome is uncertain. Process redesign requires and imparts critical skill sets. Those who lead successfully during periods of significant change usually have notable traits: they believe in and have the ability to inspire other people; they have a passion for their work and are optimistic; they are focused on a specific vision or goal and are tenacious enough to see it through to completion. They also must have the courage to make changes that may be unpleasant. In telling the story of the bear, the hospital administrator recognized the importance of facing one's fears. He began to seek a way to help middle managers cope with their own fears. Managers paralyzed by fear can rarely inspire others to make difficult changes.

Following the retreat, the administrator sought out a physician, Larry Lincoln, who is an expert in grief and loss counseling and who trained under Elizabeth Kubler-Ross. The two explored what they might do to help the middle managers work through their fears and assume accountability. They hosted a session to which all managers were invited to introduce the concept of individually and confidentially exploring their feelings about the organization's needed changes with other managers in the institution. Four groups of eight formed. Each met for eight weeks with Dr. Lincoln.

During the sessions Dr. Lincoln created an open dialogue with each group, talking about the importance of dealing with changes as if they were losses. Each individual learned that it would help to identify losses from their childhood. Such losses usually cause individuals to move into one aspect of the triangle of behavior that is difficult to break (i.e., victim, enabler, or predator). Dr. Lincoln explained that unresolved losses magnify new losses, including those experienced in the redesign of health care. To experience a loss and process it appropriately is critical to being able to move forward positively into the future. The groups, many for the first time, faced the pain of the changes they had experienced and found relief in confronting it, thereby becoming more self-assured and ready for additional change.

As the groups continued to work together they began to build a sense of community for the organization, gaining the resilience to withstand the shifting sands of the health care environment. The ability of managers to foster "reculturing" of the organization is critical and can only occur when one has learned the art. Some individuals, from their childhood, are more resilient than others and tolerate or embrace change readily. Don Berwick, from the Institute for Health Improvement, refers to the need for organizations to have both innovators and early adapters, so that timely and essential changes are embraced. For many decades the health care industry has provided a safe haven. Organizational and operational changes have come slowly, and few were forced to face their fears as they must now do.

The rapid transition to capitated contracts in managed care required that our health care system eliminate all unnecessary costs and change its way of operation. Senior leaders, concerned about the dramatic variation in the organization's ability to transform, began to search for a common model of change for the company, which would need to be global and capable of modification for all constituents. The model would serve as a common guideline, with recognizable vocabulary throughout the large organization. Several models were presented at our weekly Continuous Quality Improvement Team meetings and were evaluated for strengths and weaknesses. One model appeared to inspire and excite the group most. This model would be presented at the upcoming retreat for feedback and endorsement.

The changes that managed care has brought are as significant as those created by computer technology. It has caused providers to assume an unfamiliar level of risk and has required a true paradigm shift in how a patient is cared for and evaluated. In the hospital and in an integrated health delivery system, it is no longer enough to look at an individual department's performance. Optimization of individual departments may lead to the suboptimization of the hospital or health care system, which could be a clear path to disaster. Individual accountability must be blended with the need for common success.

Today's health care leader is responsible for understanding the organization's vision, the relationship of his or her department or area to the rest of the organization, the overall financial goals of the organization and those of one's own area, and how one's area or processes compare in cost and quality to those of the competition or those established as the benchmark in the industry. The leader must guide process improvement; therefore he or she must have statistical analysis and quality improvement skills, the ability to teach these skills to others, and the ability to advocate the changes.

LEADING REDESIGN: THE CLEAN-SHEET APPROACH

In 1993, our hospital had the motto "Team, Technology, and Tradition" and was recognized throughout the country for its excellence in patient care. But shrinking revenues, the fast-paced penetration of managed care, and the coincidental retirement of our chief executive officer of 26 years forced many rapid changes in our health care system. A strategic planning group working with the finance team studied the changing payer mix and the associated declining revenues. It realized that within the next several years, costs would have to be cut by 30% to retain the necessary margin to remain in business and to reinvest in the future.

Several departmental leaders were quietly recruited to look at reengineering their departments. The first area to be redesigned was the laboratory. This hospital system had three separate laboratory systems: a hospital laboratory; an independent, for-profit commercial laboratory; and a clinic-based laboratory originally owned by a large physician group. The executive director of the commercial outpatient laboratory was asked to spearhead an integration redesign of the system laboratories. Fortunately, there was a single pathology group for all three of the system laboratories, with a single medical director who held a clear vision for the integration of the laboratories.

The redesign effort was most challenging because there was no precedent. The first stage was to integrate the hospital lab and the commercial enterprise into a single for-profit organization, so that whether the customer accessed or utilized the laboratory as an inpatient or outpatient, there would be a common database of information and consistent and seamless services. In addition, the laboratory was asked to reduce its total cost by $800,000 the first year. The financial constraints imposed a serious redesign requirement.

Lab reengineering and the radical redesign of key processes began with a steering group of 12, including physicians, lab and hospital management, lab staff, and a facilitator. The leadership group started slowly identifying fears and barriers to change and finally building consensus around the vision for the redesigned and integrated laboratory. A clean-sheet approach was used, which has proved to be a successful tool in many difficult situations. The group identified its key customers and described what they would like each of these customers to say about the laboratory in three years. Although some of the participants had misgivings about the integration, it was relatively easy to build consensus about the ideal situation for each key customer.

Once the ideal was described, current reality was identified. The gaps between the ideal and current reality were quickly apparent. Plans for closing these gaps within a specific time period created five strategic priorities, which were assigned to specific leaders who were asked to engage six to twelve team members to create an implementation plan to reach each goal. Each team was given a set of criteria and boundaries in which to create its plan. The plans were then shared with the entire laboratory, and feedback offered by the general staff was incorporated.

In the redesign process it was clear that laboratorians, like physicians, are data driven. Anecdotal information about the need to change produced negative responses. We realized that we needed to provide specific goals to improve our result turnaround time on the Suprathreshold adaptation tests (STAT), as well as to reduce the percentage of STATs ordered at our hospital. The STAT Planning Team to some extent resisted increasing its productivity. Its members were worried about staff reductions and the loss of quality work. The facilitator of the STAT Team realized early on that the leader of the group would have to provide the team with data from other institutions that proved that the goals being set for the team were realistic. Even after providing this information, the group set more conservative goals than the leader believed possible. A year later, the data showed that the team actually beat its own performance goals by 50%. Course correction is accepted more easily when substantiated by data.

Providing the vision for redesign and the ability to remain steadfast in that vision is truly the role of the leader. Without this, most efforts will be thwarted by the many alibis for the failure of the redesign. Creating the vision is not to be equated with writing a mission statement. The vision must be both lofty and real. It will be the result of asking those in the organization to describe what they value and to what they aspire. This vision must be alive in the organization, executed with consistency and integrity. Most important, it must focus on the customer.

The leader must recognize that not everyone will board the train at the same time or place. Within a certain time frame, this should be accepted. At some point, however, not being on the train headed toward the organization's destination will require difficult decisions, which may involve some employees who were yesterday's stars but who today cannot endorse the vision of the organization. Every effort should be made to teach, retrain, and retool employees, so that they can participate. When those efforts have been exhausted and results have not been achieved, leaders must be prepared to take action, including termination.

THE OPPORTUNITIES AND CHALLENGES

Although survival in managed care requires a collaborative process, leaders must still lead. The leader sets and states the vision, initiates a process for establishing priorities and actions, champions key initiatives, and presents him- or herself as a role model for the desired behaviors. This process must be repeated every day. Senior leaders must be visible and involved in coaching these skills to middle management so that they, in turn, will model these behaviors for their staff and exhibit them to the customers they serve.

Finally, in a time when collaboration and participation are necessary, organizations often fall into the trap of treating all employees as equals. This applies particularly to the way in which leaders deal with issues of pay, rewards, and recognition. Some hospitals, because of diminishing bottom lines and implementation of teams, have eliminated merit pay, opting instead for across-the-board market increases. Instead of achieving unity and team spirit, this creates anger, distrust, and mediocre performance. It is important to reward those who demonstrate and live the values of the organization and whose work clearly supports the vision. Recognition ceremonies, both individual and team based, are very important. Tangible and meaningful rewards are essential, not just in terms of pay but for promotions, special key assignments, quality improvement team assignments, and education.

To become a successful leader in today's health care institutions, one must display creative vision, initiative and action, and the integrity, consistency, and perseverance to see the vision to fruition. Our organization is still in the throes of changing from one leadership paradigm to another. Changes are beginning to occur so rapidly that creativity and collaborative work habits are prized. Our path is leading away from bureaucracy and toward a far less structured, less formal way of working. For some this will be too uncomfortable, but for those who can make the shift, the opportunities are tremendous.

LESSONS LEARNED

The following are the lessons we learned:

1. It is important to become knowledgeable about management approaches in cutting-edge industries. Make analogies to applications in health care. This will ensure that you have a current mindset.
2. There is no substitute for true leadership. Employees expect leaders to illuminate the way, to set the course, to provide course correction and guidance, and to ensure that the key constituents are working collaboratively.
3. Timing, in a rapidly changing market, is everything. The pace of analysis, planning, and decision making must be accelerated to match or exceed the marketplace if an organization is to remain a key player. It is important to build support for major changes, but management may not have the luxury of building full consensus with all participants.
4. Timely, customer-sensitive operations require that the staff closest to the customers make many of the decisions. To do this responsibly means that leaders must educate staff about the financial aspects of the business. This takes patience and thoughtfulness to distill complex relationships and practices into a format that is clear and meaningful to any employee.
5. Not everyone can lead. One of the essential tasks of leaders is to recruit, train, develop, and promote those who are capable of continuing the leadership of the organization and its core processes.

3

Teams

Paul Bozzo

If only the world could feel the power of harmony.

Wolfgang A. Mozart

To feed a man for a day, give him fish. To feed a man for a lifetime, teach him to fish.

Anonymous

This chapter focuses on the development and roles of teams. The processes involved could be applied to any business environment because empowered, self-directed teams have many advantages. However, the concept does not provide the answer for every business seeking improved operational efficiencies. Some situations are not compatible with team formation. Any group can be composed of people with personalities that are not conducive to teamwork, or the entire group may oppose the idea of working in a team. Also, some leaders are unaware of team dynamics and are not ready to support the team concept.

The facets of team formation discussed in this chapter may help you decide if developing teams is for you. Team formation may not be worth pursuing if the employees are totally opposed to the idea. After you read this chapter, you may decide that there is nothing to gain from forming teams.

During restructuring, we at Tucson Medical Center (TMC—a hospital) and Tucson Medical Center Health Enterprise (TMCHE—a commercial outpatient lab) were on a fast track, with limited time and specific goals. We went through the merger of two labs and the reengineering process. We experienced the chaos common to most undergoing major change. During this time, we initiated team formation. The environment, saturated with change, created more fear than normally seen in a workplace. Under these circumstances, we initiated team formation and asked individuals to be more responsible and accountable.

In our efforts to achieve best value in health care, we considered teams important. They are part of the new culture that seeks and encourages fewer management positions and more independent, creative thinking. Teams set goals and, to accomplish them, fine-tune their processes. Today's leader delegates responsibilities to groups, and, as a result of dialogue with on-line employees, develops new concepts in work processes. A team creates a method to achieve greater employee involvement.

But why teams? Why not just more participation in a bureaucratic form of management? In theory, the team concept produces increased involvement with customers. The participation of those intimately involved with the processes maximizes process improvement. Theoretically, this provides greater accuracy in lab procedures and improved services, resulting in greater customer satisfaction and lower costs. Do these goals dictate team formation? No; they represent only one approach.

TEAM DEFINITION

When we think of teams, athletic teams come to mind. They have a goal—namely, winning games—and a coach who tells them how to play. The team is a group of players who choose to be there and are dedicated to winning. However, there are lessons to be learned whether or not the team wins. Being the best that you can be might not produce a win, but it is worthwhile.

Wins are the direct result of the team working together. All members must participate. Some will probably have outstanding special skills, but a team should take advantage of the special skills of all members. With their intimate knowledge of each other, teams are in the best position to maximize people skills.

Work groups are brought together to complete a specific task. Performing the task requires cohesiveness and communication. Management, not the team, sets goals and makes decisions. The opportunity exists for input but is less than that with teams. When the task is completed, the group may be disbanded. The key differentiating point is teamwork—that is, individuals cooperating to achieve goals. Teams go beyond assigning tasks to an individual. They solve problems together and have a special relationship as a team. Think of the Olympics and the special relationships formed, among the losers as well as the winners. A special camaraderie develops among team members. Teams have to communicate, in a constant and organized fashion. This may be easier to do in an industry where they work the same shift or have two overlapping shifts. It is harder in a health care environment, which operates 7 days a week, 24 hours a day.

It is worthwhile to separate work groups and teams. Defining the differences highlights some beneficial concepts, but efforts to divide groups and teams are probably not useful. There is a spectrum between the two. Teams demand much more from individuals. Team efforts are riskier and far more time-consuming. You need to analyze your situation—the personalities, the leadership, the time available, and the desired effect. Decide what works best for you. Facts in this chapter can assist you in making that decision.

TEAMS

Motivated, cohesive group empowered to make decisions
Clear team goals
Special camaraderie, commitment to other team members
Communication (structured, not random)
Team approach to problem solving
Focus on team rather than on individual performance
Continuous quality improvement, a way of life
Plans that include specifics for meeting customer expectations
Motivation and challenge
Mutual accountability
Training (interpersonal, technical, managerial, and statistical skills)

WORK GROUPS

A specific purpose, generally established by the leaders
Most approaches established by leaders
Individual responsibility
Sharing of information
Performance goals related through individuals doing their jobs

---

RATIONALE FOR FORMING TEAMS

The top management of our department—including the executive director, all the managers, and me—felt the team concept was important in achieving superior cost efficiencies in the laboratory. We wanted to form self-directed teams that would be coached, not directed. This was a new philosophy for management. We needed to value on-line employee input, and employees needed to believe that their input was valued. This meant that there had to be trust between management and employees. To achieve trust, you must "walk the talk"; that is, you must do what you say you are going to do. We were undergoing a reengineering process and felt that team members, with intimate knowledge of their processes, were in the best position to optimize their processes, improve quality, and still reduce the number of required positions, including middle management, necessary to reach our goal of a 6% cost saving in the lab.

Teams performing and knowing specific work are in the best position to take ownership and solve problems.

Prior to our involvement with teams, the nursing department had formed self-managed work teams. This ultimately played a role in our decision. Nursing's objectives were similar to ours—namely, increased quality, less middle management, and more individual involvement in the decision processes. Nursing teams appeared to be successful, but there were various levels of success.

How do you judge success? Everyone talks about measurement and outcome. We know that the team formation in nursing contributed to a decrease in full-time equivalents (FTEs) and a financial saving. Financial figures are readily available and can be used as one measurement of outcome.

Patient outcomes are frequently discussed but difficult to relate to one variable such as team formation. In the lab, cost-savings-related decreases in FTEs and patient satisfaction (surveys) where there is direct patient contact, as in phlebotomy, can be measured. You can also measure satisfaction in areas with direct handoffs (e.g., nursing and the lab). Patient outcomes can be measured as cost, functional, physical, and satisfaction (1). The lab can relate to cost and satisfaction outcomes, but it is much more difficult to relate to the other two areas, namely, functional and physical improvement. An example would be relating functional improvement to accuracy of lab tests or the turnaround time of lab results. Benchmarking to look at comparative success is questionable. It is difficult to find valid comparisons. There are some benchmarks that are similar and readily available, such as cost per test. I'm not sure if it is worth the time required to carefully relate your situation to other laboratories to achieve a comparative benchmark. In health care, your goal is zero defects. Measuring ongoing improvement (using yourself as an internal benchmark) and setting goals are always worthwhile.

We had decreased cost, testimony, and our personal observations of the quality of handoffs by nursing to the lab as evidence of nursing's success with teams. Outcome can be measured, but your intuitive sense of the quality of an operation carries significant weight in decision making. Although quality is not always easy to define, our intuitive sense of nursing's success in team formation influenced our decision to form teams.

Establishing teams seemed to be more logical than our bureaucratic structure. Teams are intimately involved with their processes, have firsthand knowledge, and should know how to fix their processes. The challenge was to make the teams appeal to the employees. We did a presentation that explained team processes; it emphasized the potential increase in satisfaction to those involved with teams, compared with working individually and reporting to a supervisor. Individual development and self-government were stressed. The concept appealed to some, but others preferred to continue in what they viewed as the easier and more secure bureaucratic methods of our past. Management made the decision for the STAT (rapid-response) lab: We would have teams. (Although team formation is best when chosen freely, in today's work environment, the decision to form teams is frequently a top-down decision. We later had other groups who chose to form teams, and their transition was smoother.) This chapter focuses on the lessons learned from our first team (namely, the STAT lab) in the hospital.

The negatives were very significant. No one had any experience with self-directed work teams, and most of the group did not want significant change. One of the nurses had been involved in forming a self-directed work team elsewhere, but the process had not been completed before she moved to Arizona. The successes in nursing were in their early stages, but we felt they were positive. We had no in-house expertise in team formation.

The lab's team formation was a learning process for management and the team members. It involved reading books, listening to tapes, attending seminars, and making phone calls for advice to the people giving the seminars.

WHY TEAMS?

Potential for: Improved productivity
                Decreased waste
                Enhanced customer service
                Increased job satisfaction

GOALS

High-performance teams are aware of and focused on achieving goals. The first step after the decision to form a team is to *find time* to set agreed-upon goals.

GOALS

Improvement in service
    Turnaround time
    Accuracy
    Correct demographics
    Decrease in the number of corrected reports
Increased involvement
    Decision making
    Customer feedback
    Problem resolution
Cost
    Improved efficiency
    Correct procedures
    Improved processes
    Redesign of work area
    Selection of equipment
    Efficient outsourcing of testing
Improvement in effectiveness
    Do the right thing the right way
    Appropriate testing
    Elimination of waste
    Fewer mistakes
    Elimination of duplication, develop synergy
    Elimination of rework
    Elimination of standing around, spread work better, flexible scheduling
Learning environment
    Technical processes
    Interpersonal relationships
    Management tools
    Statistical process

The preceding are generic goals for any laboratory or business. As with any business, more direct or indirect contact with customers will result in awareness of specific issues for resolution. The lab is no different. Simply being more involved with customers and problem resolution should improve quality continually. Prioritize customer-related goals and document them as quality improvement. The problem resolution must stress prevention. There must be an understanding of common variations that require process change, as opposed to uncommon or unusual variations. In reacting to a complaint about an infrequent or unusual occurrence, do not make changes that will solve the immediate problem but negatively affect the common processes and thereby cause even more variations. Often we are sidetracked in the attempt to put out the fire on the unusual variation and are blind to the impact on the entire process. This is less likely if the team members understand common process and uncommon variation, and work daily with the entire process.

Laboratory team goals should translate to improved accuracy and service, greater efficiency, and better cost-effectiveness. For example, improved accuracy and service would eliminate phone calls to ferret out unacceptable results, explain lost specimens, schedule redraws of blood, or request repeat testing. The improvements would save time; would provide better service, more accurate results, and greater customer satisfaction; and ultimately would save money.

We understood that we needed to improve the outsourcing process (tests sent to an outside reference lab). If quality and service were not affected and outsourcing resulted in cost savings, then we should outsource. Although this is a simple formula, it was amazing how often we had not considered the monthly send-outs to determine if we could bring additional tests in-house, cost-effectively. Moreover, the same tests were sent to different outside labs, which charged different prices for no apparent reasons. At times, the primary reference lab can send esoteric tests to specialty labs for a lower price that not is unavailable to you directly. We reviewed high-cost tests done in-house to determine their potential to be outsourced, but not as frequently as we should have.

Cost cutting was (and still is) a significant goal and driving force in the Tucson environment, which includes a large amount of managed care. If cutting costs means lowering quality, we will not survive. We must remember our role as caretakers of quality. In the long run, quality, not cost, will be the differentiating factor in health care.

LESSON LEARNED

Goals should be prioritized, periodically reviewed, and targeted for achievement in an agreed-upon time frame.

Surveys and Goals

We had the results of a recent lab survey of the nursing units from the hospital. We never prioritized key objectives, but we did share the information with the team and take action from the results of the survey.

ACTIONS TAKEN RELATED TO THE SURVEY

Share the results of the survey with nursing.

Assign pathologists to units for weekly visits.

Change print status from periodic unit reports to real-time printing (print results as they are completed).

Provide a stick-on label for the telephone that has the lab's client service number.

Show on the monitor the potential turnaround time for a test when the test was ordered (e.g., a STAT test would have the notation "1-hour turnaround time" next to it).

Change hepatitis B, lecithin/sphingomyelin ratios, and HIV run times to accommodate the labor and delivery units needs.*

Track calls from client service to the pathologists to try to ascertain if the frequency of consultations suggested underutilization of their services as consultants.

Provide normal ranges when telephoning physicians with critical results.

Do graphic turnaround studies periodically for PTT testing on the critical care units and post them every 3 weeks.

Client services, STAT lab, and laboratory information personnel participate in monthly rounds to meet the unit personnel.

*Actually, after discussions with the nursing unit, we decreased the hepatitis B testing from STAT to once per 8-hour shift, which satisfied their needs.

After reviewing the preceding listed items we came up with two obvious goals: first and foremost, faster turnaround time for tests; second, improved communication. Accuracy is always an internal laboratory goal but is assumed by customers. Not all requests from the survey (e.g., 5-minute turnaround time) were necessarily realistic, but such comments gave us an opportunity to explain some of the realities of the lab's procedure. For the hospital, we had a specific goal of a 1-hour turnaround time for all STAT tests. We tracked this for selected tests every 3 weeks for the Emergency Department and the Intensive Care units. Turnaround time was from the time the order was placed until the results were recorded in the computer.

Some events triggered a change in process. Real-time reporting of results changed the nursing unit's perception of the test turnaround time. Another example was the goal that microbiology workers not be disturbed by incoming phone calls. These calls were handled by our client service personnel, who relayed any result available in the computer. After complaints from some key physicians, we realized that the infectious disease and pulmonary specialists wanted results before they were completed and available in the computer. We decided to allow a limited number of infectious disease and pulmonary disease physicians to have the direct phone number to microbiology. We were nevertheless able to eliminate one microbiology position (FTE) as a result of the reduced number of phone calls for results.

The most effective communication remains one-on-one dialogue. Our monthly nursing unit rounds began in response to issues communicated during nursing unit rounds and by telephone. We gave a phone number to the units to use when they had problems. Problems were typed and distributed daily, as was the repeat action follow-up. The medical director (PB) and personnel from our laboratory information services, client services, STAT lab, and processing made monthly rounds to ask, "How are we doing? Any issues?" This definitely improved our image as communicators and our relationship with the nursing units. It not only gave us feedback on our goal of improved service, but provided specific issues to resolve.

OUR STORY

Management decided that our first team would be the rapid-response, or STAT, lab in the hospital. This meant letting the team make decisions on which all parties, including management, did not agree. Guidelines, however, were still required. For example, laboratory policy must conform to system guidelines. Essentially, although personnel had considerable freedom, that freedom existed only within boundaries. This is a sensitive issue requiring a delicate balance. I remember a discussion in which someone said that team boundaries needed to be more like an amoeba than a box. I agree with that. Guidelines should be relaxed enough to allow the team to work together to accomplish goals and fulfill visions, but obviously within available budget. Staying within budget and maintaining a quality operation require creativity.

Turnaround times were discussed, measured, and fine-tuned with participation from the team. Within 1 year of our reengineering, the STAT lab achieved its goal of a 1-hour turnaround time for all tests, including nonroutine ones, 95% of the time. The progress toward this goal was gradual improvement, but good data, graphed to show progress, allowed the team to witness success early in the process.

In achieving acceptable test turnaround time, process analysis, along with data on specific aspects of the process, made a difference. Justifiably, the lab is always held responsible for poor turnaround times. By taking the lead, we discovered that the delayed turnaround times were frequently related not to the technical testing but to getting the specimen to the lab. Therefore our first priority was getting the specimen to the lab promptly. The decision was made to split an FTE position with the Emergency Department. The lab employee was responsible for getting the specimens to the lab (via pneumatic tube) and for quickly tracking results when they were delayed. This significantly improved our turnaround time and image in the Emergency Department. (Since that time the entire hospital has moved to patient-care technicians who draw the blood. The lab's role in tracking turnaround time has not changed, but our primary function with regard to drawing of blood specimens is training.)

One member of the team requested a 3-month leave of absence to take care of personal business. At the time, the lab was understaffed and unsuccessfully advertising for technical positions. The STAT lab team agreed to cover for the absent staff member and employ part-time employees when necessary to fill in. Management refused, because this was not in agreement with the organization's policy. Furthermore, there was a need for staff elsewhere in the labs. Management felt that if they could spare one person, then they didn't need to add another position elsewhere in the laboratory.

Team decisions should not negatively impact the rest of the lab.

There were wage issues as well. For example, if you assume more responsibility because you are part of a self-directed work team, do you get more pay, a one-time bonus, or a mere thank you? If you give a bonus, do you link this to such requirements as attendance at meetings? Gratification at work does not come from increasing your pay a few cents. (You must feel that you make a difference.) Although the department must be market competitive, retaining a positive feeling of self-worth among employees is more important. There were potential company rewards (pay increase and bonuses) related to bottom-line improvements. However, the system was in financial difficulty, and it soon became clear that there would be no cash bonuses. The gratification would be having a position that allowed more creativity and responsibility. Because we would offer no job guarantees, the STAT lab team felt they were being exploited and they were angry. Self-directed work teams were also formed in billing and client services. With the two other teams, money was not a significant issue. In all likelihood, this was related to the fact that the latter teams were formed freely, based on a consensus of the members of the department.

Initially, there was resistance to taking responsibility. Some merely paid lip-service; a select few were volunteering. No one wanted to be team leader. With time and some initial successes, the STAT lab team began to take pride in its accomplishments. Team members divided up the workload, including scheduling, proficiency testing, maintenance, quality control, ordering of supplies, and updating of the procedure manuals.

The following indicates the status of the STAT lab team after 3 years. The team was accountable for

Scheduling: One individual was initially responsible, but this function rotated among a select few.

Procedure manuals: The process of updating and maintaining the manual was divided among the team and produced excellent results.

Hiring and firing: Members of the team participate in the hiring process. Team members interview and vote on the final decision. One person was removed from the team, which was handled by management.

Decisions: Consensus was the goal, but it was difficult to get all three shifts to participate. When consensus is impossible, the minority opinion should be acknowledged. Remember that consensus does not require wholehearted agreement with the decision, but it exists when all views are heard and all members agree to support the decision. Ideally, a decision should not reflect mere consensus but should be the result of the complete input and agreement of the whole team. A high degree of decision making should be common to all teams.

Equipment acquisition: The entire group shared in development and use of matrices for the decision process.

Technical issues: The entire group participated, resulting in agreement on selection of test methodology. There was no real debate about methodology.

Purchasing: The entire group tracked supplies and placed orders on a schedule based on supplies needed in-house.

Communication: Communication will be discussed in detail later in the chapter. Group meetings were difficult because of the small size of the team and the need to cover the lab 24 hours a day. Daily communication via a computer mailbox was successful for technical issues. There is still room for improvement in openly sharing ideas, probing, advocating, inquiring, and listening.

Education: Pathologists and technicians gave lectures that were made available on cassettes for those unable to attend sessions. The technicians who went to school to become proficient with new analyzers were responsible for teaching other team members what they learned.

The team was not fully accountable for

Budget process: The budget process is not fully resolved; discussion is ongoing. Budgets are distributed regularly, and attempts at one-on-one education with representatives of the group have been unsuccessful. At the time of this writing, a team leader position was developed and filled. This person, not the team, is responsible for presenting the budget status on a monthly basis.

Decision process: The decision process has worked well with minor decisions. Major decisions, such as flexible scheduling and process changes, did not fully materialize. This is primarily due to lack of scheduled group time, which contributed some unwillingness to take the responsibility individually.

Performance: Peer participation in a 360-degree evaluation process was established, but the team was not involved in coaching. This was not done regularly, but we were hoping to provide candid, constructive feedback. We were definitely moving in the right direction.

Disciplinary action: Disciplinary action is still inactive after 2 years.

Customer relationships: For the most part, customer relationships have been left up to the team leader and pathologists.

Conflict resolution: Conflict resolution has worked with minor conflicts, but major conflicts were never resolved by the team.

Participation: Most participated in team activities, but not everyone.

We are not perfect in any of these categories, but we are constantly improving. Teams are a way of life for us, and, like life, they seem to involve a journey rather than an end.

Strategic Priorities

With the participation of team members, strategic priorities or critical success factors were developed for the entire lab, including the STAT lab. Strategic priorities should result in a plan for getting from where we are to a future goal.

- We would operate as a single lab, which is (and is perceived as) the best-value lab. There would be convenient rapid lab services for physicians that were easily communicated, timely, and accurate.
- We would build teams across the lab with a common purpose and vision. Participation of a cross section of the laboratory in this process was intended to give a sense of "we" for the entire lab.
- If we were to create a single, merged lab, then we needed *standardization* of methods, equipment, quality controls, normal values, critical values, and reporting formats.
- We would develop seamless, hassle-free laboratory services for patients and physicians. This meant working toward convenience and accessibility. Goals for external customers (physicians, nurses, office staff, appropriate hospital staff) include one call for any laboratory result, computer hookup, and a data repository for the doctors.
- Technical personnel would do the technical work, and personnel at lower-paid positions would do the nontechnical work. Processing of samples (e.g., separating the serum from the red blood cells) had been done in sections by the technical staff. But, in keeping with this strategic priority, the phlebotomist's role was expanded to include entering patient demographics and preparing or processing the specimens. Initially, some of the technical staff resisted because this change meant loss of control and fewer technical positions. We worked hard to identify the number of FTEs necessary to perform the work efficiently and cost-effectively. The system leadership had decreed that savings of $800,000 would be generated from the laboratory. It was obvious that this could not be accomplished by merely defending old processes, keeping the same FTEs, and working faster.

These priorities are just as significant today as they were when they were established, but like all strategic priorities, they should periodically be reexamined and recommunicated.

Top Leadership Role

Self-directed teams have a unique arrangement with management. They are part of a system and must respond to its boundaries. Administrative hierarchy will continue to exist and need not be threatened by team formation. Management maintains a role that includes coaching, mentoring, providing resources that include training, and, in general, supporting the concept of teams. Management should run interference and help overcome major obstacles, but the team needs to identify those obstacles. Team-related quality measurements shared with leadership are a means of tracking progress.

Leaders need to do more than stand on a mountaintop shouting down such directives such as, "Have goals, form teams, communicate, solve problems." Leadership must assist the team in developing clear cut goals and purposes. This doesn't mean that the leaders will create the goals. Leaders should arrange for meetings where team members share ideas on goals and ways to improve job performance.

One of the problems remains knowing when to let go of the reins and get out of the way. Why do managers have a hard time with this? It is difficult to give up control and to feel less needed. Giving the teams responsibility and accountability, which varies with the make-up of each team, is a balancing act. An important factor is commitment to the team concept. If you delegate responsibility before the team is ready to accept the resulting accountability, it can be a disaster. Some teams may form with little help from management, but that is the exception. More often, top leadership functions like a symphonic conductor who coordinates the work of all the players.

A good leader steps aside so that other leaders can emerge from these teams. But leadership involves more than just letting it happen. You must help it happen, make it happen, and at the same time promote this as a team effort. This is no different from other continuous quality improvement groups. You should ask, "What are your goals? How are we going to achieve them? What resources are needed? When will this be accomplished as judged by measured data?" Coaching is one of the crucial roles for management in relationship to teams.

We had received a directive to form teams, but we had a reluctant technical group, and some members of management feared that improved efficiency could cost them their jobs. Some believed that teams were a fad and wouldn't last. Although there were small victories along the way, it took about 1 year to show significant progress. The results indicated improved turnaround time, increased workload, and positive feedback from customers. This was accomplished by adding responsibility, employing fewer FTEs, using attrition rather than layoffs, and allowing the team to make decisions. Results were the fuel that improved morale and attitude. Acknowledging team success is critical, but too often ignored.

"As for the best leaders, the people do not notice their existence.
    The next best, the people honor and praise. The next, the people fear; and the next, the people hate. When the best leaders' work is done the people say, 'We did it ourselves.' "

Lao-Tzu, Chinese philosopher

LEADERSHIP'S ROLE

Foster team performance.
Delegate control to the team.
Remove major obstacles.
Be aware of the quality of the operation.
Drive fear out of the workplace.
Coach.
Mentor.

Need for Team Leaders

All teams need a leader. With the added responsibilities, the person who acts as a leader will not spend as much time performing lab tests. Team leaders work as part of the team but delegate as much as possible to create self-management or self-direction. Some recommend rotating team leaders, but not all team members possess leadership ability. Those who succeed are persistent, have the ability to delegate, and bring the team together to make decisions. Reading books or attending courses on team leadership can help but may not be enough. The leader's goal is to maximize team performance.

The following are some of the attributes required:

Has the desire to lead.
Is a communicator and has above-average listening skills.
Knows and understands the system's purpose.
Delegates, creates opportunities for others.
Helps clarify the roles of the individual.
Focuses on the process, not the people.
Knows how and where to find help.
Works well with management.
Has meeting skills.
Is persistent in moving toward desired goals and establishes measurements to show progress.
Does real work, including some of the less desirable tasks.

It is an exceptional team that has multiple people with leadership abilities. It is even more rare when all team members are capable of rotating this position.

Selecting the Groups to Form Teams

We formed multiple groups, not necessarily self-directed work teams, with each representing a different work area. The groups at the hospital were STAT lab, processing, and microbiology; the core lab represented a fourth group that was further divided into technical, processing, phlebotomy, client services, marketing, courier, and billing. Of these groups, client services and billing would form self-managed work teams. Why these three teams? Forming the STAT lab team was a management decision, whereas the billing and client services teams were group decisions promoted by management but not dictated by it. The STAT lab was a merger of hematology, urinalysis, coagulation, chemistry, and special chemistry. Management felt this radical change would be facilitated by forming a team that would participate in designing a new area, changing processes, and selecting new equipment. By supporting a STAT lab team, management felt it would send a message on participation, responsibility, and accountability.

Client services and billing referred to themselves as a work-centered team, in which skilled, well-informed people take direction from the work itself rather than from management.

Process Review

The leadership was unwavering in its demand that the process be improved. Once you encourage change, processes should continue to be revisited. Make this a periodic agenda item for meetings. Sharing responsibility for reagent preparation between shifts and performing maintenance during slow periods were changed over time. Process steps that didn't add value, such as microbiology computer screens, were gradually eliminated. You must continually ask, "Why are we doing this?"

With the help of neutral facilitators and some management, processes were reviewed by the STAT lab team. The key was redesign. With modular lab furniture and movable analyzers, the team was able to try different configurations until the design of the lab was optimal for moving specimens. Although this started with a step-by-step analysis of the testing process on butcher paper, the critical portion (the redesign) was done entirely by the team using practical trials as the last step before finalizing a decision. This and retooling (new equipment selection) were real team efforts. For equipment selection, we created an extensive matrix that included the cost of reagents, frequency of calibration, time to make up reagents when necessary, quality controls, technical time for test performance, required maintenance, bar coding, costs of either owning or leasing the equipment, and many others. We realized that we had too many vendors for equipment, reagents, and quality control. Our goal was to have fewer vendors, standardized reagents, better quality control, and equipment that not only would reduce costs, but would allow for uniformity of testing results from multiple sites.

Bringing in outsiders to help analyze the process would have encouraged more change by showing us a different perspective. For example, a physician or nurse as an outside lab process analyzer might suggest that they receive part of a test earlier rather than wait for all the results (e.g., get the automated portion of a blood count rather than wait for the manual differential); if there is insufficient serum to run an entire group of tests, the unit should be called and asked to help select the more critical tests.

The key is commitment to do what is necessary to make the operation lean without waste. If the intent is there most teams will figure out the rest on their own.

Training

Training is an important, but frequently neglected, part of team development.

Training was the weakest part of our program. We brought in several people to talk about team development, but we did not have much time and did not offer training in many of the skills needed. We realized that training in interpersonal skills, management, and statistical process was available in our system, but we did not have sufficient extra staff to allow personnel to attend these courses. Consequently, we struggled with trying to acquire these important skills gradually.

Training must be ongoing and constantly repeated, for old habits are not easily broken. Technical training was provided by the vendors, the pathologists (quality control), and individuals who had gone to school for instruction on individual pieces of equipment. Management needed to understand the budget—total costs, cost per test, and other financial terminology, because these were used to measure team performance. We needed training in statistical process to review and process quality improvement data.

We had several one-on-one sessions on budget with volunteers from the STAT lab, but this information was not communicated to other members of the team. We are continuing to supply the data and offer assistance in understanding budget. The lab's chief financial officer gave some general lectures on the topic and offered to review the data one on one with any member of the STAT team. The system offered courses on statistical processes, but no members of the STAT team participated. Budget was an issue for our entire lab. This was resolved for the entire merged lab when sections rotated presentation of their financial status at the weekly management meeting.

We trained one of our client service employees in statistical process, and she now provides periodic data on turnaround time for key nursing units and other information as needed. Requests for specific information came primarily from nursing unit rounds and a problem log. The clinical rounds were made monthly by the medical director, personnel from the laboratory, system information systems, client services, and the STAT lab. The extensive time commitment was such that the STAT lab did not consistently participate in rounds until a team leader was hired. The problem log was compiled from calls made to a phone number set up specifically to record issues from the clinicians, nurses, unit clerks, and other customers. These were answered and recorded in the log in a timely manner. We summarized these problems regularly, looking for trends that would become goals for quality improvement.

Self-management

How far do you go with freedom of choices for self-managed, self-directed, or work-directed teams? There are appropriate boundaries to define the latitude within which the team will work. These latitudes will be different for each organization but are defined by the system and the abilities of the group. Hierarchy remains in place. Self-management does not imply the absence of management; rather, it involves the creation of a different role. Some of the boundaries will be defined by the team (e.g., the degree of involvement with budget). Policy changes are subject to approval, but every effort should be made not to negate team decisions.

A Lesson to Be Learned

I continued to make decisions without consulting the team. I thought they were small decisions, but the team resented them. For example, I decided to bring Tegretol testing back to the hospital from the outside core lab. We had originally decided to send certain low-volume (less than 12 per month) tests to the core lab. The decision was based on the clinicians' original willingness to tolerate a 2-hour turnaround time. All these tests were higher-volume procedures in the core lab. The physicians in the Emergency Department were unhappy with the Tegretol turnaround time. Even though they agreed with the economics, they really wanted the results in 1 hour. Though we averaged only 10 tests a month, I decided to return the testing to the hospital without consulting the team. The STAT lab team should have participated in the decision. I agreed that I was wrong in overstepping decision boundaries and promised to be more aware and try to improve my communication in the future.

LESSON

Little actions that come from top management send a big message.

Communication

You must share information if you are to evaluate ideas and improve job performance. We had weekly meetings, but sometimes they were merely gripe sessions. At times, problems were resolved, but personnel issues, such as vacation and benefits, detracted us from discussing such items as the work processes, division of work, and responsibilities. Human resource issues, although important, should be kept separate from routine team meetings. In the initial stages of team development, I would suggest that wages, benefits, performance, and competence issues be reviewed and dealt with by the team and the Human Resources Department as separate issues.

We had the usual ground rules for meetings, such as the following: stay focused on purpose, listen, do not engage in side conversations, participate, start and finish on time. We had a ground rule about staying focused, but we should have defined the purpose of each meeting more clearly. It would have been helpful to spend the last 5 minutes of each meeting discussing how effectively we had used the time.

With 7-day-a-week, 24-hour-a-day coverage, attendance at the meetings was poor. We held the meetings at different times and in the STAT lab, hoping for better participation. At times, we covered the lab with part-time employees so that the full team could participate in the meetings. We should have done this more often, but per diems were not always available.

QUALITY MEETINGS

Stay focused on the purpose.
Follow ground rules.
Set goals, solve problems.
Set dates for completion of specific goals.
Review accomplishments.

We posted meeting minutes and asked personnel who attended to take the information back to their co-workers and discuss it with them. These efforts met with limited success. Team dialogue required a presence. Well-organized meetings of all personnel periodically allow for minority views that may not be expressed by representatives. With full participation, the bottom line will be more representative and frequently different.

- Total team participation in the meetings was necessary.
- Attitude impacts communication.
- Communication requires respect.
- Good listening skills must be developed.
- Posting minutes keeps the contents of the meetings more consistent than word of mouth.
- Some daily form of communication, such as lab computer mailbox, is important.

Because everyone had to sign on to the computer each day, one of our most successful tools was the computer mailbox. This does not develop dialogue, but it does allow for timely communication.

Communication of the team with direct handoffs and other customers is as important as internal team communication. Teams do not work in a vacuum, and there are always handoffs. As mentioned earlier, clinical rounds and our problem log were effective in changing the image of the lab. The lab was frequently cited at system management meetings for aggressively pursuing customers' needs.

Better communication means better listening on the part of everyone, including management and team members. Listening skills can be developed, but not without the desire to be a better listener. Once that occurs and you truly try to understand what is being said, you overcome a major hurdle.

Here are some basic rules for improving communication.

- Don't think about what you are going to say until the last person has finished speaking.
- Try to understand the speaker's position.
- Stay focused on one topic at a time.
- Rephrase periodically what has been said to make sure you understand.
- Keep eye contact.
- Say things as plainly as possible.
- Use visual aids.
- Speak for yourself, not for others.
- After a position is advocated, start inquiries with who, what, where, when, and how.

Sharing data is a necessity for every team. Healthy communication produces critical feedback and improved performance.

LESSONS LEARNED

The following are some lessons we learned:

1. Teams are not the solution for everyone.
2. There must be a true commitment to being a team.
3. Top leadership must strongly support the team concept as exemplified by their actions.
4. Have a mission and specific measurable goals.
5. Have both long-term and short-term goals.
6. Be persistent with regard to goals.
7. Periodically review short-term goals.
8. Be sure that goals have a date for completion.
9. Remember that it is best to start with a team leader.
10. Set up initial rules and boundaries.
11. If the team concept is not acceptable to an individual, try to move that person to a different position in the system.
12. Provide ongoing training.
13. Remain involved and accountable for the process. This is the way to optimize learning.
14. Expect periodic frustrations from team members.
15. Establish a relationship between the team and customers.
16. Focus on process improvement and getting rid of waste.
17. Identify specific waste.
18. Be data driven, and measure improvement.
19. Remember that meetings are absolute necessities, but if poorly run they are worthless.
20. Communicate (listen, listen, listen).

CONCLUSION

A significant impediment to team formation may be that decision makers do not know how or when to develop teams. Teams are not the solution to every problem. Goals requiring minimal change do not need teams. Key attributes of successful teams are positive for every organization. This includes more accountability, increased production, decreased waste, and greater job satisfaction, with resulting decrease in absenteeism and turnover. This can be done with top-down management and work groups, but the achievement may not be as great. A significant drawback to high-performance teams is the time required for development. Work groups still need to have clear goals, look at their processes, and improve their communication. However, finding the time necessary to develop team skills may not be realistic.

In many cases, leadership will play a major role and facilitate greater participation and achievement of desired results, such as decreased waste. Success will vary with the skill of the leader, just as team success will vary with the skills of the members.

STAGES OF TEAM DEVELOPMENT

Forming: Cautious, guarded team affiliation.
Storming: Competitive, strained work relationships.
Norming: Harmonious cohesiveness.
Performing: Collaborative teamwork.

In a study of teams looking at defined stages of development, the authors concluded that most teams are complex and that vestiges of stages remain. High-performance teams are not common. Part of their uniqueness is their commitment to each other. Most teams never achieve optimal performance as seen in a study of Fortune 500 companies (2).

We should try to develop as many of the positive attributes of high-performance teams as possible. Too often lack of full group participation prevents us from achieving high-performance teams. We did not have full participation from any of our teams, even though it may have seemed so on the surface. However, a good deal was accomplished using the team processes. More important, we achieved a feeling of "we" throughout the entire lab, and the desire to work toward optimizing customer satisfaction by fulfilling their needs.

In the new model of getting things done, teams build strong relationships. People, not technology, are our most important asset. Building interpersonal relationships is one of the most important and most difficult facets of organizations, whether in team formation or in top-down management. People are more valued in the team model whether it is a high-performance team or merely a group of people who work well together. However, not having a high-performance team does not mean solo efforts or suboptimal performance. Start the team process and be selective in your efforts; aim initially for small wins. Continue to learn and improve while always striving for the goal of a high-performance work team. Team formation is one way of achieving accountability and pride in your work. We do not have high-performance teams, but we have team accountability and pride. We have achieved our major goals and continue to strive for improvement. We hope that our story will result in a more cohesive workforce and a better lab for you. No one knows why great teams come together or how to replicate their magic.

What we want, regardless of our process, is people coming in every day looking for a better way to do things.

REFERENCES

1. Nelson EC, Mohr JJ, Batalden PB, Plume SK: Improving healthcare, part 1: The clinical value compass. *J Qual Improv* 1996;22:243–256.
2. Montebello AR: Teamwork in healthcare: Opportunities for gains in quality, productivity and competitive advantage. *Clin Lab Manag* 1994;8:91–104.

4

Evaluations

Paul Bozzo

To laugh is to risk appearing the fool.
To weep is to risk appearing sentimental.
To reach out for another is to risk involvement.
To expose feelings is to risk exposing your true self.
To place your ideas, your dreams before the crowd is to risk their loss.
To love is to risk not being loved in return.
To live is to risk dying.
To hope is to risk despair.
To try is to risk failure.
But risks must be taken, because the greatest hazard in life is to risk nothing.

The person who risks nothing, does nothing, has nothing, and is nothing.
He may avoid suffering and sorrow,
but he simply cannot learn, feel, change, grow, love, live.
Chained by his certitude, he is a slave, he has forfeited freedom.
Only a person who risks is free.

Author Unknown

WHY EVALUATE?

Evaluation involves critique. Critique exposes. Exposure is a risk. Evaluations optimize improvement, and the gain outweighs the risk. If we were to survey a large number of institutions, we would find that most performed evaluations. They may be called appraisals or reviews, but they fall into the same category, namely, a performance review of an individual. The significant issue is whether they are worthwhile. In theory, they are an opportunity to look at areas of improvement that will increase your individual growth and make you more valuable to the system. If that were consistently the perception by those being evaluated, none would consider debating their worth. In fact, evaluations are all too frequently an annual written opinion of the supervisor, who may or may not know much about you, and generally has been remotely involved with your work. But the job description of supervisors includes writing appraisals or evaluations. All too frequently, the person being evaluated would say that it was a waste of time. Evaluations are used to judge performances with an attached stick and carrot. Do well and you may get a bonus and keep your job. Do poorly and you may not get a bonus or may even lose your job.

A good evaluation challenges you, supports you, helps you realize your potential. If the evaluation were all flowers and roses, you might love it, but it won't challenge you to grow. You cannot learn to walk if you are not willing to fall. No risk, no reward.

You may encounter the desire to eliminate evaluations altogether. When done properly, evaluations can be used as an opportunity for dialogue. If nothing else, they will bring to light rumors regarding the process.

Ideally, a summary of a 360-degree evaluation (in which fellow employees and customers participate in the evaluation process), a self-evaluation, and a final appraisal by the evaluee should be reviewed periodically throughout the year. It is valid to question doing this only once a year. Has there been communication throughout the year, and in what form? The evaluation will be better received if personnel believe the evaluation involves no monetary rewards and is truly for self-improvement. An example of compensation criteria used to calculate a bonus would be using scores on problem solving, initiative, teamwork, and customer service. Supervisory requirements can be used to calculate 40% of the bonus, whereas quantity of work and technical expertise may be used to figure 60% of the bonus. Kohn argues that incentives can be perceived as punishment: Succeed and you are rewarded; fail and you are punished by no increase in compensation (1). The same applies to plaques, employee of the month, and so on. The argument against this form of recognition is that long-term growth is sacrificed to short-term returns. These are all poor substitutions for genuine interest in job, system, and self-growth. Many measured gains are related to team, not individual effort. Despite the level of performance of individuals on teams, market performance of the organization remains the critical factor for many monetary incentives. Some organizations place the employees at risk if the company does poorly. Some argue that employees cannot control the market and therefore should not be placed at risk. Others reply that the process ties the employee into company goals and that they should take risks if they are to also expect to gain.

I have been involved with three or four different evaluation formats. Some were used to determine whether the employee received a bonus or raise; others were not. I favor the latter because I believe that the value is self-improvement and not financial reimbursement. Unfortunately, if we are to maintain incentives, finance is a sensitive area and is still used as a reward for a positive performance. With the financial pressures on health care, many still feel it is their only available source of incentive. This is unfortunate because a job well suited to individuals, in which they feel they make a difference, is a key motivational factor. The recognition of good performance is part of leadership's responsibility. Phony praise for the sake of praise is not worthwhile, but positive statements that are deserved remain invaluable.

In reality, if an employee continues to receive poor evaluations from his or her fellow workers and supervisor, chances are his or her job would be in jeopardy, most likely as a consequence of specific issues outside the evaluation. We need to reemphasize that evaluations ideally are used to improve performance and perceptions of self-worth.

The real dilemma is how leadership can do this without creating an adversarial relationship with the employee and at the same time creatively give something of value back to him or her. Performance appraisals are a necessity, but they can be done in a positive manner. Unfortunately, in times of restructuring and downsizing, evaluations are frequently used to determine whether or not an employee remains with the system. Therefore fair performance appraisals are absolutely necessary.

Edward Deming, one of the pioneers of quality improvement, felt that pay was not a good motivator. He felt strongly that evaluations were a cause of fear that should be eliminated. It was one of his key 14 points (2).

> Make the environment such that the average person feels that growth is his or her number 1 objective.

GOALS

Goals that are specific, attainable with effort (stretch goals), and measurable are ideal. Vague goals are less likely to be achieved because they do not focus on specific tasks. Goals may be personal or professional, but they frequently overlap. If you are in sales, it is easy to create a measurable goal, such as the number of new accounts or new revenue generated. But even these formulas can be fraught with problems. For example, what if those sales result in a negative bottom line? Should you get credit for the related gross revenue? Theoretically, in the field of medicine, we try to relate achievement to patient outcome. Outcome is multifaceted and includes much more than mortality and morbidity (3). Just because a patient dies, it doesn't necessarily mean that we should be downgraded. We may have done a great job with the care of the patient. Quality of life and dignified death are reasonable goals, but two of many. A more appropriate and encompassing goal should be customer satisfaction. Satisfaction includes social, functional, medical, and economic factors (4). What is crucial is that the patient and family feel that everyone is making an honest effort to do their very best to promote a positive outcome for the patient. Frequently this kind of information is only available through surveys. Surveys involve significant subjectivity. The personal interview surveys may prejudice the answer by the wording of the question, the tone in which it is asked, or the body language of the surveyor. They should be done by professionally trained personnel, not volunteers; unfortunately, in the health care industry volunteers are often used. Questions should be clear, specific, and not aimed at a specific answer. The entire survey should be concise. Time spent learning and understanding the science of surveys can result in better future use of this important tool. The laboratory is sometimes viewed as only remotely connected to patient outcome. However, accuracy, service, correct test utilization, and cost all affect patient satisfaction.

Individual Goals or Team Goals?

Goals often can be measured using information available through the computer, including financial data, diagnostic service utilization, and ICD-9 codes (diagnostic code for test used to determine appropriateness). This is difficult information to relate directly to an individual performance evaluation. Cost of testing is better related to teams. For example, an ideal objective would measure the lab's contribution to the system goals but still allow measurement of the performance of individuals or specific teams. Some potential goals for individuals or teams are as follow:

Team Goals

Improved turnaround time for specific tests and specific areas, such as partial thromboplastin times in the coronary care unit

Customer service (turnaround time, communication, dependability, etc.)

Reduced cost per test

Individual Goals

Cross-training on additional instruments

More in-depth understanding of quality control

Improved interpersonal relationships

Goals of Pathologists

More appropriate testing by developing consensus with clinicians

More in-depth knowledge of specific areas

More continuing education in subspecialty area that would improve the group's overall performance

More time spent teaching (e.g., continuing education)

Fewer variations on peer review

GOALS

Developed with input from associates or team, and shared with others who can offer assistance

Resources needed

Obstacles

Plan

Specific and easily understood by any two reviewers

Measurable

Challenging, so that people can invest themselves more fully in their work

Achievable in the current reality

Established in writing, covering specific time periods

Structured with flexibility to respond to the environment

Used to help create job satisfaction

Reviewed periodically

Goals must be in writing. Establishing milestones serves as a reminder and makes the objective more achievable. This demands periodic appraisal of the status. You cannot have milestones if the goals cannot be measured and are not achievable. Personal goals include better interpersonal skills, being more of a team player, and being more sensitive to the feelings of other team members. These are reflected in listening, being open to suggested changes, and showing respect to other individuals. Failure to listen carefully is frequently viewed as a lack of respect. Goals related to learning may require developing a study habit to improve your skills or spending more time teaching. Teaching, which allows give and take with the participants, always improves one's skills.

One objective measurement would be the number of education hours related to your job. Physicians must take a certain number of continuing education hours every 3 years. If this requirement is fulfilled, does this make you a more knowledgeable and better physician? Certainly not, but it does constitute a requirement that can be measured objectively. And it is a step in the right direction. However, those who are best at taking courses and tests are not always the most caring individuals, nor do they always have common sense or good medical judgment.

Schools have been discussing the merit of evaluations for years. Grades create a fear factor used to sort students for future education or job opportunities, but they do not provide positive feedback when the student is doing well. Furthermore, they should be used to promote coaching when the students need improvement.

The most difficult challenge is getting personnel to treat development of goals as something of value to them rather than a chore. Frequently, in response to a discussion of goals, I hear statements like, "I just want to do my job." Moving toward an objective occurs only when that goal is continually examined and when one also examines how close one is to achieving it. What coach would mention winning a game against an arch rival and only go over it once? What would be the chance of winning a game without a game plan?

Taking the time to work out these goals is worthwhile. All too often, goal setting is done hastily and with minimal commitment. Of what value is a general goal, such as, "I want to be a better person," or, "I would like to be a more knowledgeable pathologist." Be more specific. Any goal, if achieved, helps you feel better about yourself and is worthwhile. Perhaps your goal is weight loss or working out more. These can be listed as personal goals. Three to four goals are recommended. There is no perfect number, but start with at least one goal and continuously fine-tune it.

Do you have a passion for something in your work? Are your goals tied in with that passion? If they are, there is considerable pleasure in achieving them. The goals that we choose freely without any compulsion are critical. We excel at the things we want to do. Are your business and professional goals achieved only because the situation demands it? If you have no passion for excellence in your job, should you continue to work in that field? If you cannot develop any worthwhile goals, what does it say about the journey you call life? What is your destination? The satisfaction of improving on who you are and your work is worthwhile. The lack of this in your life can be detrimental to your well being. We spend a major part of our waking hours at work, and it should be a positive experience. Time spent examining goals may be helpful in changing not just your job, but perhaps your life.

TEAM GOALS AND PERFORMANCE

As we examine processes in the lab, we begin to realize that many goals can be achieved only by a cooperative effort between groups of people not necessarily limited to the lab. The lab does not work in a vacuum. Many handoffs affect service and cost issues. Team goals should be reached by a team consensus. These goals should be sensitive to customers' needs. Improved turnaround time for laboratory tests is an example of goals that can only be accomplished by a team. Another example is the quality and time required for the surgical reports. Each of these examples requires examining the efficiency of handoffs to other departments. Clinicians do not remember that one pathologist is faster than another, but they remember the slow turnaround time for a few of the many surgical reports. They remember department performance; they do not necessarily remember the individuals involved. If the department does a great job completing the surgical report but the results never reach the chart, the clinician does not view this as good service.

It is essential that team members and customers participate in the process. Don't wait for criticism to develop a team goal. Communicate and learn what your customers expect. Then get creative and dazzle them.

As with any criteria to judge performance, existing forms should serve only as guidelines and should be adapted to the circumstances in which they are to be used. Achievement of team goals is part of the evaluation process.

TEAM GOALS

Shared risks
Shared accountability
Shared reward

Performance Criteria

It would be helpful to eliminate subjective terminology such as *average, excellent,* and *good.* Alternate terminology, such as *needs improvement, not a strength, meets expectations, a strength,* or an *exceptional skill* are better but still mean something different to everyone. At the least, grading specific performance criterion gives you a consistent comparison with a group of peers. Scoring allows you to see trends in areas of performance, especially when compared with previous evaluations. The trend is more important than the individual scores of a specific question. Deal with the criteria that are important to the system and are customer centered. Review interpersonal skills as well as technical performance. Evaluations should not be limited to technologic competency. We want to identify efforts and achievements that are below *acceptable* or *meets expectations.* These are areas for discussion, coaching, and potential improvement.

Do not forget to focus on the positive aspects of the evaluation. Frequently, all that is remembered are the negatives.

Quantity should not be ignored, but all quantity is not equal (e.g., processes not performed at a high level of quality).

An important aspect of a team or individual evaluation is that all individuals share the workload. Frequently, this is the only criterion that is used when looking at quantity of work. Quantity, as reflected by schedule, does not always reflect reality (e.g., the medical technologist who is skilled mechanically and is called on whenever there is equipment to be repaired, or the pathologist who does more consulting on difficult surgical cases). Generally, this is not reflected in the evaluation. Adjustments or specific comments for such situations are of value.

Evaluation of an individual's interpersonal skills (listening, conflict resolution, and so on) is an extremely subjective, sensitive, and important area. Very few jobs are limited to working alone. If you work entirely out in the field, customers should participate in the evaluation. Other issues include integrity, trust, respect, and confidence. If these are missing, it is difficult to build solid working relationships. Integrity develops trust. Do what you say you are going to do. In addition, you must be competent to gain respect and confidence from your associates. You can become more competent if you recognize and correct areas that can be improved. This is the true value of evaluation. For most, interpersonal skills generally can be improved with coaching.

In a work environment, it is easy to perceive certain patterns in your fellow workers that interfere with good working relationships. These include complaining without being constructive, avoiding problems, being unwilling to take responsibility, having poor communication skills, and most commonly, developing listening skills. Does listening mean waiting your turn to talk? What if you listen, agree, and do nothing different? This will be interpreted as poor listening, indifference, or, even worse, arrogance or passive-aggressive behavior. Everyone has an opinion on whether or not a fellow worker is a good listener. Everyone has a view of a fellow employee's ability to resolve conflicts and solve problems. If an employee doesn't deal with problems or avoids them, then he or she cannot demonstrate problem resolution, and this is a true deficit. Knowledge of this should be valuable input to someone who is trying to improve. Do you really want to work in an environment where someone doesn't care what you think of your working relationships or where someone doesn't want to improve his or her interpersonal relationships? Fear of such exposure prevents the necessary risk taking to undergo the evaluation process.

Interpersonal relationships (where such qualities as trust, respect, caring, and listening are demonstrated) are extremely important to all evaluations and worth reemphasizing. They contribute to the environment that allows us all to work most efficiently. An angry co-worker can make you less productive because you become frustrated or angry and therefore work less efficiently. I remember one worker who prompted three other people to tender their resignation. You don't want that attitude in your environment. The situation was honestly discussed and resolved. But for some time issues were avoided and communication was poor. This occurred 20 years ago, and coaching, mentoring, and team were not discussed. These situations demand immediate attention and should not be postponed until the annual evaluation.

Once you decide on performance criteria, you must establish how they will be communicated to the employee and define management's role in tracking, mentoring, and coaching. Unlike judging, coaching is a mutually constructive situation. A good coach helps you improve, has suggestions on overcoming deficiencies or obstacles, and offers praise for positive achievements. Compare this with coaching sports. If the sport is football and the problem is tackling and the coach doesn't know much about it, he or she sends you to someone with expertise in that subject. The same principle applies to business coaching.

Another competency that you might consider scoring is initiative and amount of supervision required. If employees have initiative, they recognize what is needed and can go beyond what is assigned without being asked. They initiate improved ways of doing something and are active in the process. Some people need infrequent supervision and only seek a supervisor when needed. At times, employees are intimidated by the supervisor and are unwilling to show initiative because of a history of supervisory repercussions when this occurs. If an entire group lacks initiative, this could indicate that a supervisor is responsible.

All these parameters of performance should be discussed by the group, ideally including those who are to be evaluated as well as some outsiders. An outsider with previous experience in evaluations can add a different viewpoint. Develop performance indicators appropriate to your environment. In general, discussions of interpersonal skills are confrontational. One's motives for such a discussion are questioned, and fear may inhibit any examination of the skills in question. Evaluations are generally done because someone in authority (e.g., a top-level system leader) has decided they should be done. It is rare that a group chooses to undergo evaluations. The evaluation is an opportunity to explore these areas in a positive fashion. Because it is uncomfortable, there may be resistance to the process. But the potential gains are significant. Total acceptance comes when the recipient perceives personal value as a result. Emphasis on the positive and assistance in planning positive improvement will change beliefs about evaluations.

INTERPERSONAL SKILLS

Trust
Respect
Caring
Listening
Problem/conflict resolution
Initiative

Productivity

Goals for productivity in the health care field are seldom useful as a stand-alone item. Without computer-generated data, collecting results related to productivity can be time-consuming. We can easily obtain computer-generated data on costs and other objective numbers, including number of tests. If anatomic pathology is computerized, it may be possible to count the number of surgicals, outside consultations, fine-needle aspirations, slides, and variations on peer review for pathologists. Always include a denominator in any peer review number. Five variations out of 100 are more significant than five out of 1,000. For the quantity to be valid, there should be some data on the complexity of the cases or tests in surgical pathology. You could have a system that assigns surgicals where you merely describe the gross appearance (e.g., orthopedic hardware) as one unit and complex cases as four units. Simple cases, requiring few microscopic slides and little time (e.g., a gallbladder), could be given two units. The cases between two and four are assigned three units. This will help define complexity. This system is fairly simple, but given a large number of cases, it will give you some idea of the case mix. To be worthwhile, ratings should be done consistently and for a significant period of time.

A problem with pathologists' productivity is accounting for the pathologist who is the most frequent consultant of the group on difficult cases. You could create a field to track intragroup consultations. If we were to sit around, have a cup of coffee, and have an honest discussion, we would know who does the most work, who is more quality-oriented, and who interfaces more with the clinicians and the clerical and technical staff. Unfortunately, egos, fear of financial implications, and personality traits get in the way. You could end up with subjective data that could be over- or underrated. You could also track consultations, problem resolutions, and projects in clinical pathology as well as anatomic pathology. This would be extremely time-consuming and impractical. If you do this, each area should be defined. If you participate for 10 minutes of a 2-hour meeting, are you really participating? Possibly, but your contribution would have to be significant. Just being present does not qualify you for participating. Every phone call is not a consultation. This may need to be limited to consultations that you formalize with a written report. For many groups, this change would eliminate tracking consultations altogether, because informal consultations are the rule.

The data are more complex than just looking at a number for productivity. You should include data on the quality of the work for a more valid look at productivity. I don't know of any worthwhile system that addresses this. Basically, most pathology consults are acceptable (e.g., surgicals or hematology differentials) and only draw attention when criticized by the clinician or when they are at variance with peer review, outside consultations, or clinical diagnosis. Like beauty, productivity is in the eye of the beholder. It is something each person knows when he or she sees it and is perceived differently by everyone. We are going to live with the concept of productivity or quantification of work; therefore we should try to make it as valid as possible. The only area of the laboratory with any consistent production is cytology, and this is related to imposed regulations.

Quantitation and quality production for phlebotomists would have to consider difficult draws. Obviously, you would like to define *difficult draws*, but this is not easy. What is difficult for one might be easy for another, more skilled person. Who teaches the other phlebotomist? Who is called when there is a difficult draw? Personnel are aware of this person's abilities, but this is not taken into account when reviewing productivity. Because such a person may do the most difficult draws, he or she may have the most repeat draws. Look at the number of repeat draws or the number of contaminated blood cultures over a period of time by a particular phlebotomist. Other factors of value are availability (i.e., the phlebotomist who is always available to work when someone doesn't show), the ability to resolve problems, and time spent teaching. Excessive tardiness and absenteeism over a long time period (more than 6 months) is worth monitoring. Most systems have, or should have, standard guidelines in this area. Slight but repeated tardiness is not only unfair to fellow workers, but generally seriously irritating. In addition, data on the individual phlebotomist garnered from patient surveys or body substance precaution adherences are beneficial (see the appendix). When you decide on the categories, you can track them prospectively. Discussions of this nature need to take place after the last evaluation so that measurements can be in place for future evaluations.

> Discussion of the evaluation process can be of considerable value in preparing for future evaluations.

Pathologists

The appendix lists representative duties of pathologists and medical directors that could be converted to questions and used in performance evaluations. They should be scored by peers who are knowledgeable about these activities. A scale from 1 to 5 or 10, should be used. You should also have categories called *don't know* and *not applicable* with each question. Have an area for comment below each set of questions. This may be more valuable than the actual score. Again, response trends from groups of questions are more important than the individual scores.

Management

Objective numbers such as net revenue, number of tests, costs per test, or adherence to budget indicate nothing about such key attributes of this position as vision, creativity, ability to promote teamwork, motivation, coaching, mentoring ability, and positioning for the future. These are all valid points that are both extremely important and subjective (see the appendix criteria for management evaluation). These criteria should be reviewed, critiqued, and finalized with the input of others in the process.

Note that these same management criteria will apply to the medical director. (See appendix.)

Customer service requires turned-on people: It's hard to be turned on if you are not supported by management.

Medical Technologists: See appendix.

Microbiology

A. Peddecord et al. published a microbiology survey based on input from infectious disease specialists. This reflected quality for both team and individual leaders. Overall quality was rated on a scale of 1 to 5 (with 5 being excellent), with individual scoring for bacteriology, mycology, mycobacteriology, parasitology, and serology. A list of types of problems and approximate frequency per year included the following: quality of consultations with microbiology supervisors and directors; mishandled cultures; inability to recollect culture; inconsistent culture diagnoses among microbiologists; failure of lab to call critical clinical results; lack of clarity of reports necessitating calling the lab for clarification (5). This is an excellent example of the use of surveys to solicit customer input and points out potential customer-related goals for a section.

Couriers

Specific issues for evaluation include quality and timeliness of vehicle maintenance, specific complaints, and traffic records. Customer satisfaction, interpersonal effectiveness, teamwork, and system–value alignment should also be rated. Willingness to contribute in an exceptional way should always be noted. For example, one courier drove 160 miles to rescue a disabled vehicle, deliver reports, and pick up test specimens after she had finished her normal shift. This level of commitment deserves special recognition. Comments from specific clients regarding individual couriers are always worthy of praise and should be placed in the individual's file. We had one courier who, survey after survey, received comments from clients such as "a real pleasure to work with" and "the best." This was from our annual lab survey of key customers that was not courier focused.

We don't want evaluations to be police actions, but any past disciplinary issues serious enough to warrant action must be considered when summarizing evaluations and should be recorded in the employee's file. Evaluations should show improvement from year to year. Serious issues that continue to surface on a regular basis require coaching and mentoring. If the situation does not improve, then perhaps a change of work environment should be considered.

What your boss, your peers, and your subordinates really think of you may sting, but facing the truth can also make you a better person.

Self-evaluation

A self-evaluation can be an important part of the process (see the appendix). An initial self-evaluation would list personal goals. The goals should be specific, measurable, achievable, and compatible with the system and departmental objectives. Periodic reappraisal of progress allows one to acknowledge either a poor process or a lack of commitment. If a self-evaluation is done annually, it should include an honest assessment of the progress toward the previous year's goals. The evaluee may want to review his peer evaluations before writing a self-evaluation. An alternative is to draft a self-evaluation describing your objectives; then do a review with input from your peers. If necessary, they can reprioritize, add, or delete certain goals. Too often we are only willing to look at our successes that are easy and ego stroking. It is too painful to look at failure, but this is exactly why the same mistakes are made repeatedly. Achievement of goals specified in a self-evaluation is worth reviewing.

In general, we are our own best critics. It is amazing how often an individual may know what the issues are and even want to change but have no plan of how to do it. Self-assessment is a great starting point for self-improvement. Taking the time to reflect quietly on your self-image—who you are, where you are, where you are going, and where you would like to go—is always worthwhile and seldom done. What image would you like to project? This is an example of why psychologic therapy without a crisis can be so worthwhile. "Every day, a bit wiser" is a reasonable goal, but it requires looking back and deciding what we've learned about the world and how we got to where we are today. I'm not suggesting that we live in the past, but that we use the past as instruction for the future.

Does the individual have a purpose in his/her work and in life? Is work meaningful? What bothers a person about work? Are there areas where he or she would like to be more involved? Is the person aligned with the system? Although it is true that the system should have a core ideology to guide individuals, each person's purpose will be unique. If the individual finds the ideology of the system unacceptable, this is a red light not to be ignored. Can the individual influence the institution's ideology, or should this person consider another company? Successful companies don't and shouldn't easily change core ideology. It may be time to say, "This is not a job I want or should have." It may be worthwhile to attach the system's and departmental vision to the self-evaluation.

Evaluators should not only consider areas for improvement but provide positive feedback as well. Try to be specific and constructive. The same applies to the evaluee. I have coached individuals with outstanding evaluations, including a large number of peers who are obsessed with a few constructive criticisms. Make this a rule for evaluators: Come up with at least one positive. If they are done correctly, 360-degree evaluations will improve team relations.

If something in your relationship is bothersome, give a specific example and suggest how the process could be improved to correct the issue(s). In the future, this will result in dialogue related to a specific incident occurring in a timely fashion, not limited to the time of evaluation. The real goal is more open and honest communication, performed with sensitivity.

Additional evaluation forms are listed in the appendix and may serve as a model for your forms.

360-Degree Evaluations

Some people look at evaluations as an opportunity to be critical and forget that they are meant to bring out the positive as well as the negative. A wise old song states, "Accentuate the positive." In a 360-degree evaluation or feedback, the evaluee selects six to eight (or any agreed-upon number) colleagues (internal customers) or external customers from whom to solicit feedback. Internal customers are fellow employees who interact with the evaluee or are in a position to observe him or her regularly.

I endorse the team approach for evaluations. Evaluators can choose to remain anonymous but should be selected from peers and be able to provide a true 360-degree evaluation. This means participation of fellow workers, including multiple authoritative levels from the organization. This is a customer-focused approach and therefore should include not only fellow workers (internal customers) but also external customers. The person being evaluated can submit a list of potential evaluators but should not exclude those with whom he or she works closely. This would include any person in a direct supervisory role. It is easier, but less profitable, to look only at favorable evaluations.

Timing

Doing all the evaluations in the same time period is time-consuming. The effort applied and quality of the evaluation may be related to how many have been completed that day. An alternative is to spread evaluations throughout the year, utilizing the anniversary date of employment. Unfortunately, for most systems, timing is related to financial incentives, which may be tied to the fiscal year. The 360-degree evaluation seems to be more accepted if all are done simultaneously within a deadline. If all are done at the same time, it provides a better atmosphere for critique of the process for the future. An additional advantage of the annual shared time for evaluation is that the evaluators will be reviewing multiple individuals with the same process, resulting in more consistent comments about a group of evaluees.

The Evaluation Summary and Interview

Several options are available in the evaluation summary and interview, and each has its pluses. The evaluee can write a letter explaining the need for the evaluator's input, with the comments returned directly to the evaluee. This requires maturity from the evaluee and is the ideal. But evaluators may feel intimidated and fear some form of retribution. The evaluations can also be returned to a neutral party or could be anonymous. Nevertheless, even if the comments have no identifying source of origin, the person being evaluated can frequently discern the source from the pattern of the comments. In my experience, the comments have almost always been given anonymously, and this is the approach I favor.

The comments are the primary focus of the evaluee's attention, but consistently low or high scores for individual questions are significant and indicate a trend. Furthermore, a comparison with others may be significant if everyone else has scored high but the individual being evaluated has consistently scored low. Multiple sources would indicate a valid score rather than just an individual's biased view. For example, if you have six evaluations that are scored on a scale of 1 to 5, a perfect score would be 30. Thus your score on that would be circled but you would also be able to see how your peers had done on that particular question. Except for your score, the other scores should remain anonymous. This approach is a response to the comment that everyone gets the same score on this question.

It is hard to escape the perception that we are policing the individual, and that is the last thing we want from an evaluation. Providing the data without comment may be worth considering, especially if used uniformly for that group and with foreknowledge and consensus of the group on the data collected. It is valuable to let the individual know how he or she compares with peers.

You can also graph the response to see how you compare with your peers. (See data from Aurora Health and HPSA.) (Fig. 4-1)

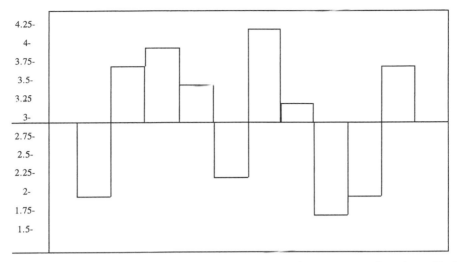

FIG. 4-1. Pathologist evaluation by supervisory personnel shows concern for others. Each bar represents a different pathologist. Control limits equal two sigma. Also see appendix page 81.

FINAL SUMMATION

Unless the evaluation forms have been mailed back to the individual, give the evaluee the information from the evaluations anonymously and ask him or her to assess their impact, discussing both positive and negative results. Regardless of the manner of distribution, the information should be reviewed by a coach. Does he or she feel that there are concerns worth working on as a result of this input? Ask the evaluee to construct a plan for realizing the potential positive changes, and be willing to document and discuss them. The action plan should reflect not only the result of the 360-degree evaluation, but also progress on objectives from the individual's previous self-evaluations or personal objectives. It is harder to be adversarial with one's self-evaluation or a group of comments than with comments assumed to be from one individual. If multiple people come to the same conclusion, is that not an indication of the validity of the issues?

In business, the previous guiding motto was, "If it ain't broke, don't fix it." More significant today are two facts: (a) we can always improve a process, and (b) we need to look at what we're doing right, and do more of it. This can be traumatic, but the goal is to make it worthwhile because it results in self-improvement.

I have had the responsibility of writing evaluation summaries on my own, getting input in writing the evaluation, adding self-evaluations, going to a 360-degree evaluation, giving all the data anonymously, and finally having the evaluee review the data and write the final evaluation with all data in hand. At the time of this writing, we are discussing the option of giving evaluations directly to the evaluee. This helps avoid an adversarial role with the coach or mentor. I have seen horrible bottom lines of evaluations result in unreal rationalization because criticisms are not seen as opportunities. Thus evaluees go into denial and an adversarial situation may be unavoidable. Time may improve the situation. Ask for reassessment in 3 months; you may want to do more than one evaluation process in a year. This final question should be asked if it hasn't already been addressed by the evaluee: "Knowing what you know now, what would you do differently?" Employees themselves are the best source of the cause of poor employee performance (4).

Evaluations should appraise not merely how you follow, but how you lead. This may sound strange, but successful companies are made up of those who feel that what they think and do is important. This does not mean that they are not team players; to the contrary, creative thinking is what makes a team effort worthwhile. Otherwise, we might as well have dictatorships. Some managers are threatened by creativity and potential. They might see an individual in a different light when he or she is evaluated by an entire group.

ADVICE FOR THE FINAL SUMMARY

Listen first and talk later.
Emphasize employee development and performance.
Do not give personal feedback.
Be specific.
Emphasize observable employee performances.
Be positive first and if necessary negative later.
Ask opened-ended questions, beginning with *what, how, when,* and so on (3).

Moving Toward Self-improvement

Evaluations are an opportunity to stimulate the evaluee to grow into what he or she wants to be. A common theme suggested recently has been, "I want to be more involved in a management role related to cost-saving matters." This is fine, but it only works if you have a plan. It is not enough to sit around and wait for an issue to surface so that you can participate. We have to walk the talk. Lech Walesa, in addressing the United Nations said, "We have heard enough words." This is so true. Back up your goals with an action plan, and if it is not working, seek help. The evaluation process can be painful. We need to make it a positive force, so the evaluees perceive it to be of value to them.

RELATIONSHIPS AT WORK

Positive	*Negative*
Trust	Avoiding
Respect	Overreacting
Affection	Complaining
Confidence	Lecturing

Listening Skills
Stay focused, want to listen
Ask thought-provoking questions
Bring out touchy subjects
Encourage people to talk more

LESSONS LEARNED

The following are some of the lessons we learned:

1. Have challenging definitive written goals.
2. Performance standard:
   Have input from participants.
   Include interpersonal issues.
   Whenever possible, have specific and measurable goals.
3. Use a 360-degree evaluation involving fellow workers at all levels.
4. Have the individual being evaluated do a self-evaluation, write his or her own summary of the evaluation and plan for improvement.
5. Review goals periodically.

HIRING PRACTICES

Having gone through evaluations and realized that some individuals seem poorly suited to their position, logic should lead you to examine why you hired that person in the first place. If we are to succeed and people are the key ingredient, then hiring practices must be reexamined. The process of hiring is subjective and frequently superficial. The goal should be hiring an individual who contributes to your system and your individual department's goals. You must focus on getting the right person for the right job.

Application

The application should provide adequate information, including job history. Personal references listed are generally positive and contribute little. Professional references, such as previous supervisors, are frequently worthwhile. Check all references. A phone call is generally better than a written reply. Written replies can be vague. Tone of voice or a hesitation can be as significant as the spoken word. Professional background checks, including Social Security records, may show frequent moves and any criminal record.

Interview

The prescreening may be done by a team, but not necessarily one limited to participation from the section where the applicant would work. Using areas outside the job-specified area, where there are handoffs to that position, provides different views of the applicant's response to situational questions. Situational stories and the applicant's reaction to a dramatized role are worthwhile and give some perception of involvement in his or her potential work role. Focus on attitude toward previous employers and fellow employees. Try to elicit their response to potential problems. They should know something or want to know something about your organization. For examples of interview questions see the appendix.

Necessity of the Position

In this era of cost containment, we must decide if you need the position. Consider the following point:

1. Is this a replacement position?

2. What would be the impact to service, quality, and cost if this position is not filled?
3. If this is a new position, will it improve the bottom line in excess of salary, benefits, and other expenses?
4. Have you benchmarked your department costs?

Evaluations emphasize the need to fine-tune hiring practices. Too often they are not given the attention needed. In this day of team/customer focus, it is a mistake not to find new hires who will fulfill the organizational needs, including both technical and interpersonal skills. Market-value salaries are a necessity to acquire quality personnel. The most important part of the organization is people. Hiring is the most important thing you do as a leader.

CONCLUSION

The debate on the value of evaluations will continue. Results will also be used to determine compensation. Whether this is positive or not is questionable.

Evaluations that contribute to individual growth and promote positive performance are worthwhile. Evaluations used correctly are a tool for self-improvement. For many companies, even if the policy is well designed, implementation in a positive manner is the challenge.

PRIORITIZED REASONS FOR EVALUATIONS

Self-improvement
Coaching
Training/development
Compensation
Retention

REFERENCES

1. Kohn A: Why incentive plans cannot work. *Harvard Bus Rev* 1993;(Oct-Sept):54–63.
2. Deming WE: Out of crisis. Massachusetts Institute of Technology, Center for Advanced Engineering Study, 1982.
3. Goodale JG: Six steps to improve discussions of employee performance. *Clin Lab Manage Rev* 1995;9:7–14.
4. Nelson EC, Mohr JJ, Batalden PB, Plume SK: Improving health care, part 1: the clinical value compass. *J Qual Improv* 1996;22:243–256.
5. Peddecord KM, Baron EJ, Francis D, Drew JA: Quality perceptions of microbiology services: a survey of infectious diseases specialists. *ASCP* 1996;105:58–64.

APPENDIX

Representative Duties of the Pathologist
1. Maintains high standards of practice in anatomic and clinical pathology.
2. Renders consultation to clinicians utilizing and correlating laboratory data (clinical and anatomic pathology) for diagnosis and patient management.
3. Supervises and is responsible for medical activities in Anatomic Pathology and Clinical Laboratory in conjunction with Medical Director and laboratory management.

4. Is knowledgeable about regulatory requirements and ensures laboratory compliance.
5. Is involved in new test selection and development, equipment selection, timeliness of reports, and interpretation of test results as needed or requested.
6. Participates in ongoing process that ensures complete current procedure manuals that are technically followed.
7. Stays current with scientific advances in specialty areas.
8. Attends meetings and shares that information.
9. Participates in teaching for resident staff, medical staff, and laboratory staff on a regular basis.
10. Attends staff meetings and accepts and actively participates in administrative committees of the system and/or laboratory.
11. Works with management in recruitment and maintains top-quality laboratory technical and clerical staff.
12. Participates with managers in strategic planning, setting goals, and developing and allocating resources and budget planning appropriate to the medical environment.
13. Responds to reported problems/incidents in a timely, effective manner; investigates and evaluates changes needed to avoid future reoccurrence. Recommends appropriate change where indicated.
14. Supports and promotes departmental/hospital safety programs; assists in ensuring that section complies with safety policies of department and accrediting/regulatory agencies.
15. Provides assistance and demonstrates active understanding in initiating and monitoring quality-control/quality-improvement activities, including appropriateness of testing and clinical pathways involving the laboratory participation.
16. Reviews and evaluates proficiency testing results of his or her assigned section(s); assists the supervisor in ensuring that these results fall within acceptable ranges, discrepancies are investigated, and corrective steps are taken and documented.

The preceding are the more traditional areas of concern for pathologists. Here are some additional potential performance criteria for pathologists:

Creativity in maintaining state-of-the-art laboratory
Performance as a team player, including willingness to listen and flexibility
Number of surgicals, including number of slides and/or cases, possibly quantitated with a weighted score for difficulty of cases
Evaluations done by customer, including multiple physicians from different specialties and others that they hand off to, such as nurses
Quantity and significance of variations found on peer review
Quality of intradepartmental consultations
Knowledge and support of system goals
Willingness to accept and experience growth related to constructive criticisms

Depending on the design of the position, many performance characteristics overlap with those of the pathologists. In addition the following should be considered.

Representative Duties of the Medical Director
1. Assumes professional, consultative, organizational, and administrative responsibility (shared with the Executive Director) for the laboratory services.

2. Is responsible for implementing and maintaining the regulatory standards.
3. Interacts with the pathologists, physicians, patients, administrators, and other employees. Demonstrates good communication skills.
4. Provides direction and leadership in implementing and monitoring standards of performance involving quality control, quality improvement (including pathology peer review program), and cost-effectiveness of the laboratory, including ancillary services (e.g., point of care testing). The quality improvement program should interface with all services involving lab handoffs.
5. Is responsible for ensuring that there are sufficient qualified personnel with adequate documented training and experience to supervise and perform the work of the lab.
6. Participates in and involves others in goal setting, developing, and allocating resources appropriate to the medical environment.
7. Is involved with budget planning and control with responsible fiscal financial management.
8. Provides educational direction for the medical and laboratory staff.
9. Participates in and is responsible for the selection of qualified reference laboratories.
10. Promotes a safe laboratory environment.
11. Is responsible for an interface with clinicians regarding the appropriate selection and interpretation of laboratory test results.

Potential Criteria for Management Evaluation

Customer focus.
Builds credibility by acting as a role model who demonstrates commitment to values developed by the system and those in it.
Demonstrates commitment and inspires others to commit to system goals.
Structures environment to allow employee participation in goal formation.
Communicates goals.
Achieves objectives supported by a good planning process, including periodic measurement and reevaluation of actions.
Encourages others to help, individually or as a team, with planning and problem solving.
Organizes work in an orderly fashion.
Recognizes good performance.
Controls details.
Delegates appropriately.
Is approachable.
Builds a team spirit.
Tries to make work stimulating and interesting.
Helps foster good morale.

Representative Duties of the Medical Technologist

Demonstrates commitment to quality by providing accurate results.
Participates in activities requiring responsibility beyond the usual duties, including scheduling, proficiency testing, maintenance of key equipment, supply coordination, and accountability for a quality improvement monitor.
Participates in committee work.
Number of test reports corrected. (An example of the potential problem would be working with equipment that had functioned correctly in performing the control tests and then malfunctioned, which produced erroneous results. This may have been impossible to detect. Also many test processes may be initiated by one technician and com-

pleted by another. Only the last technician would be listed by the computer as the responsible individual. Thus, these corrected reports, at times, may not reflect individual effort. Nonetheless, over an extended period of time, trends may surface.)
Understands and correctly applies quality control.
Participates in continuing education.
    Education sessions given.
    Education sessions attended.
Misses as few workdays as possible.
Is seldom tardy.
Is creative. (This is somewhat vague, but people with creative ability are extremely important to the future of any organization. This sometimes means thinking beyond the normal confines. It is a skill that is not necessarily natural, but it can be taught.)

Interview Questions

A nurse calls and accuses the phlebotomist of being rude to a patient. How would you handle the situation?
You pick up a specimen at the doctor's office and are told that a report from a surgical biopsy submitted 3 days ago still has not been received. What is your response?
What is your definition of *leadership*?
Give an example of a problem or conflict resolution in which you have taken the lead.
You're new on the job and you're given directions to do a specific task. However, you don't feel the process is efficient. What is your response?

Customer Service

1. You have an angry customer calling and demanding results. Results are not ready. How do you respond? (Does this person have the skill to diffuse angry customers, and will he or she take the initiative to research the status of the specimen? If he or she feels the process could be improved, how could that be done?)
2. How do you assess the needs of your customer?
3. What is customer service? What do *you* expect as a customer?
4. Describe a situation where you have experienced exceptional customer service. What about the interaction made you feel good?
5. Describe a situation in which you felt you did not make your customer happy. What could you have done differently?
6. A physician's office calls for specimen requirements of a test you are unfamiliar with. You realize it may take a few minutes to get the information. Describe the steps you take. Will the caller be placed on hold or be called back? What data will you use to make that decision?
7. A patient calls about an x-ray. She seems confused and has trouble describing what she wants. Your services do not include x-rays. What do you do?

Team Participation

1. Describe a situation where a decision was made that you did not agree with. (Did this person speak out? If so, did the person support the decision and respect the difference of opinion?)
2. Have you ever been in a situation where you found mistakes on someone else's assignment or area of responsibility? What did you do? What would you do if the mistakes were chronic?
3. If a co-worker does something that you do not agree with or hurts you in some way, what do you do?

4. When do you feel it is appropriate to speak about a co-worker with another co-worker?
5. Describe a situation where you did not care for a person you worked with.
6. Are you familiar with working as a team? Describe your role as a team member. What made it a team and not just an individual effort?
7. What experience have you had with motivating others? Yourself?

Additional Interview Questions

1. Tell us about yourself and why you are interested in this job.
2. What do you know about TMCHE/TMC laboratories?
3. Please describe the range of your current responsibilities and the relationship you have with other leaders at NW Hospital. Please describe the boundaries you have in terms of hiring new staff, purchasing equipment and supplies, and changing processes.
4. What do you know about patient-focus care, and what do you know about the successes others have had in implementing it in their hospitals?
5. What kinds of quality improvement teams have you led? Participated in?
6. Have you ever had to make a decision before you had all the data you wanted? Please give an example. What did you do?
7. Has a policy or directive come down with which you really disagreed? What was it? What did you do?
8. How much stability would you like in terms of a fixed job description? How much have you had at other organizations?
9. Do you feel that the chain of command is important? Why? When do you feel it might inhibit organizational effectiveness?
10. What responsibility do you have for budgeting? What budgeting method do you use?
11. Give us an example of something major you have done to save money for your organization.
12. How would you describe your management style? How would your employees describe it?
13. What was the style of the best manager you have worked for? What did you learn and begin using from that person's approach?
14. What do you enjoy most about being a manager? Least?
15. How often do you think it's necessary to meet with your employees? What do you talk about?
16. Have you had to manage a personnel situation with a potential legal impact? Please describe what your role was and what you learned from it.
17. Have you had to make oral presentations to other managers? Describe them.
18. How do you assess priorities? How do you assign them?
19. Give us an example of a change you saw coming, or something you thought was necessary to change. How did you go about planning for it?

TABLE 1. *Phlebotomy Survey*

Dear Patient:

As a valued customer, your opinion is not only important but critical if we are to continue efforts to provide quality services. With this in mind, please take a moment to complete this survey and return it to TMCHE Laboratory.

1. Did the phlebotomist identify him- or herself? YES NO
2. Did the phlebotomist explain the procedure? YES NO
3. Did the phlebotomist appear neat and clean? YES NO
4. Did the phlebotomist appear skilled at drawing blood? YES NO
5. Did the phlebotomist make you feel comfortable about the procedure? YES NO
6. Did the phlebotomist protect your privacy as a patient? YES NO
7. Would you allow the phlebotomist to draw your blood again? YES NO
8. Did you wait long? YES NO
   If so, how long? _____

What can we change to give you greater satisfaction? Please be specific.

_____

Comments:

_____

_____

TABLE 2. *BSP (Body Substance Precaution) Survey*

Date: _____

Section: _____

Monitor initials: _____

Title: BSP protective gear

Criteria	Yes	No*	NA
1. Gloves are worn when touching blood, body fluids, mucous membranes, or nonintact skin.			
2. Gloves are worn for handling items or surfaces soiled with blood or bloody fluids.			
3. Gloves are worn when contact with blood is possible (IV initiation, fingersticks, etc.).			
4. Gloves are worn when policy or procedure requires them.			
5. Hands are washed immediately after gloves are removed.			
6. Gowns or aprons are worn when there is potential for blood and/or body fluids to splash onto the caregiver.			
7. Masks, eyewear, and/or face shields are worn when policy or procedure require them.			
8. Protective facewear is worn when care is likely to generate droplet or splashing that could expose the mucous membranes of the caregiver.			
9. Protective gear is available for use.			

Title of person being observed: _____

  *Document noncompliant activity and follow-up action for each response in the "No" column on the audit.

_____

_____

_____

TABLE 3. *BSP Survey*

Date:				
Section:				
Monitor initials:				
Title:	BSP sharps disposal			

Criteria	Yes	No*	NA
1. All used needles/syringes contaminated with blood/body fluids are placed uncapped in the sharps box immediately after using.			
2. When used needles/syringes must be recapped, a recapping device or a one-hand technique is used.			
3. All sharps from patient procedure trays are placed in the sharps box immediately after a procedure is completed.			
4. Sharps disposal boxes are not overfilled and are properly disposed of when full.			

Title of person being observed:

*Document noncompliant activity and follow-up action for each response in the "No" column on the audit.

TABLE 4. *BSP Survey*

Date: _____

Section: _____

Monitor initials: _____

Title: BSP infectious waste disposal

Criteria	Yes	No*	NA

1. Appropriate equipment/resources are available for use for container or infectious wastes disposal (autoclave bag).
2. Equipment and supplies (bleach and spray bottles) are available for use on blood or body fluid spills.

Title of person being observed: _____

*Document noncompliant activity and follow-up action for each response in the "No" column on the audit.

_____

_____

_____

TABLE 5. *BSP Survey*

Date: _____

Section: _____

Monitor initials: _____

Title: BSP handwashing compliance

Criteria	Yes	No*	NA

1. Washes hand after emptying wastes and/or container.
2. Resources available for washing hands (soap, paper towels, sinks—all convenient)

Title of person being observed: _____

*Document noncompliant activity and follow-up action for each response in the "No" column on the audit.

_____

_____

_____

TABLE 6. *Aurora Health Care Laboratory Services pathologist evaluation by clinicians*

Please evaluate for the following attributes and return in the enclosed envelope by _____ . If you are unfamiliar with this pathologist, please check here _____ and proceed to the next evaluation.

Please choose only one box at the right per question

	Rarely	Some-times	Fre-quently	Almost always	Don't know
1. Is courteous.					
2. Is friendly.					
3. Is readily available for reviewing pathology or cytology cases.					
4. Is readily available to solve problems relating to the clinical laboratory.					
5. Is willing to solve problems relating to the clinical laboratory.					
6. Is quick to respond to your questions or problems.					
7. Follow-up, when necessary, is done quickly.					
8. Follow-up, when necessary, is satisfactory.					
9. Instills confidence in his or her medical knowledge.					

Suggestions for improvement

_____

_____

_____

_____

_____

_____

TABLE 7. *360 Degree Feedback*

360-DEGREE REVIEW FEEDBACK RECEIVER: _____

Feedback supplier (circle one):   self   coach   colleague   direct report   other

	Virtually always	Rarely	Some-times	Often

CUSTOMER SATISFACTION Answer only for observed behaviors

FOCUSED ON CUSTOMER NEEDS

	Virtually always	Rarely	Some-times	Often
Listens to understand customer's point of view	☐	☐	☐	☐
Follows up with customer to ensure needs have been met	☐	☐	☐	☐
Reliable/dependable in completing tasks and commitments to customer	☐	☐	☐	☐

FRIENDLY

	Virtually always	Rarely	Some-times	Often
Courteous, pleasant	☐	☐	☐	☐
Is positive when interacting with others	☐	☐	☐	☐
Shows care and concern for others	☐	☐	☐	☐

FLEXIBLE

	Virtually always	Rarely	Some-times	Often
Handles multiple assignments	☐	☐	☐	☐
Adjusts to changing situations and needs	☐	☐	☐	☐
Seeks win/win in meeting customer needs	☐	☐	☐	☐

FAST

	Virtually always	Rarely	Some-times	Often
Is timely in meeting customer needs	☐	☐	☐	☐
Corrects mistakes quickly	☐	☐	☐	☐
Provides accurate, appropriate service the first time	☐	☐	☐	☐

INTEGRITY Answer only for observed behaviors

DEMONSTRATES HIGH ETHICAL STANDARDS

	Virtually always	Rarely	Some-times	Often
Exhibits honesty in actions and in decision making	☐	☐	☐	☐
Displays fairness in dealing with others	☐	☐	☐	☐
Is truthful in interacting	☐	☐	☐	☐

TRUSTWORTHY

	Virtually always	Rarely	Some-times	Often
Makes and keeps promises	☐	☐	☐	☐
Does not speak negatively about others	☐	☐	☐	☐
Apologizes when appropriate	☐	☐	☐	☐

MATURITY

	Virtually always	Rarely	Some-times	Often
Is honest and forthright	☐	☐	☐	☐
Displays maturity in interactions and in decision making	☐	☐	☐	☐
Accepts constructive criticism and assumes responsibility for improvement	☐	☐	☐	☐

TABLE 7. *(Continued)*

	Virtually always	Rarely	Some-times	Often
PEOPLE Answer only for observed behaviors				
PROFESSIONAL EFFECTIVENESS				
Seeks out and participates in learning opportunities	☐	☐	☐	☐
Shares job knowledge readily with others	☐	☐	☐	☐
Strives to balance personal and professional goals	☐	☐	☐	☐
LEADERSHIP EFFECTIVENESS				
Regularly provides others with constructive feedback and contributes to others' development	☐	☐	☐	☐
Takes time to coach or mentor others	☐	☐	☐	☐
TEAMWORK Answer only for observed behaviors				
ACHIEVING MUTUAL GOALS				
Works together with teammates to accomplish desired outcomes	☐	☐	☐	☐
Demonstrates commitment to team goals; holds accountable for team effectiveness	☐	☐	☐	☐
Contributes as an equal member of the team	☐	☐	☐	☐
SYNERGY				
Seeks out others' points of view	☐	☐	☐	☐
Demonstrates support of teammates' accomplishments	☐	☐	☐	☐
Avoids placing blame on others	☐	☐	☐	☐
WIN/WIN				
When dealing with conflict, strives to find solution that benefits all	☐	☐	☐	☐
When dealing with conflict, confronts the issue directly with the individual involved	☐	☐	☐	☐
Respects every individual in every interaction	☐	☐	☐	☐
PROCESS/OUTCOME Answer only for observed behaviors				
CONTINUOUS IMPROVEMENT OF PROCESSES				
Suggests ideas for improving the way the job gets done	☐	☐	☐	☐
Openly accepts suggestions for individual improvement from others	☐	☐	☐	☐

TABLE 7. *(Continued)*

	Virtually always	Rarely	Some-times	Often
Contributes as an equal member of the team	☐	☐	☐	☐
QUALITY/COST BALANCE				
Continually strives to improve timeliness, accuracy, and quality of outcome	☐	☐	☐	☐
Shares ideas for cost savings	☐	☐	☐	☐
INNOVATION				
Suggests ideas for new or enhanced products or services to satisfy customer	☐	☐	☐	☐
Displays imagination, creativity, and resourcefulness in satisfying customer needs in a cost-effective manner	☐	☐	☐	☐
ACHIEVEMENT				
Consistently accomplishes objectives and takes on extra tasks as necessary	☐	☐	☐	☐
Accepts full accountability in accomplishing tasks/projects	☐	☐	☐	☐
Takes pride in work	☐	☐	☐	☐
KNOWLEDGE/SUPPORT OF ORGANIZATIONAL GOALS				
Demonstrates understanding and support of organization's culture, purpose, and values	☐	☐	☐	☐
Understands how individual duties support the organization's mission	☐	☐	☐	☐

Feedback supplied by (optional): _____

List facts to be shared with the receiver to substantiate feedback above. (Additional sheets if necessary.)

_____

_____

_____

_____

_____

_____

5

Cost Analysis in the Laboratory

Neil R. Lautaret and Paul Bozzo

We have used various financial analysis tools and processes over the years to measure performance and set goals for process changes and improvements. Some of the lessons learned are illustrated using an integration process that merged our reference laboratory and our hospital laboratory. The two laboratories were both owned by the same parent but for the last 10 years had been operated separately. Our goal was to integrate the two laboratories, with a rapid-response laboratory in the hospital and a core lab concept for all other testing.

Since our initial integration, we have applied financial tools to measure and internally compare performance and to review opportunities to work with potential partners. The goal of this chapter is to present a financial approach that will save time and help create consensus. Cost analysis and financial comparison are crucial in the day-to-day operation of the business, benchmarking, or any potential merger. Obtaining valid comparative data can be easy if the tools used are kept simple and the users agree to measurements that are consistent, are user-friendly, and can be benchmarked with other institutions. These are important factors to consider when selecting and implementing financial tools to evaluate your business.

NEED FOR A GOAL

During the merger we had a financial goal dictated by the need for the laboratory and the system to have a positive bottom line now and in the future. The goal should dictate not only direction, but also the required time for completion. Our first integration was guided by a mission statement with goals of quality, service, and savings of a specific dollar amount within 1 year. Many financial evaluations of projects are attempts to determine profitability. Calculations for return on investment must consider future reimbursements. Net revenues (gross revenue minus deductions) have decreased significantly in most markets as a result of capitation (payments per member per month) and cutbacks in government reimbursements such as Medicare and Medicaid. Capitation will not be limited to managed care (HMOs, or health maintenance organizations) but has already begun with other payers, such as Blue Cross/Blue Shield. The financial implications for the future are the same whether you are part of a large system or an independent laboratory. In retrospect, revenue decreases in our laboratory occurred faster than anticipated. We were in an environment of shrinking revenues; if we had continued to experience a negative bottom line, we would not have survived.

After much deliberation at the executive level, we were mandated, along with the rest of our integrated health care system, to reduce expenses 8% from the prior year. We now had a target that was real. We would be the first department in the system to move forward using reengineering or rightsizing. In our case, and for most systems, this meant downsizing. This dollar amount represented reality to the laboratory employees. It was a goal that they could grasp, was measurable, was not an option, and required real change. To our employees, just saying, "Reduce costs" was too vague; they needed a dollar amount, which was meaningful and provided a tangible goal that would affect the decision-making processes.

CREATING A GOAL

If your goal is not mandated, then create a realistic one for yourself. One method is to consider a percent of something such as gross revenues (gross charges), net revenues (gross revenues minus revenue deductions such as write-offs), last year's expenses, or net income (net revenue minus expenses). Using a percent may skew the data. If your net revenue base decreased as a result of an outside factor such as a higher percent of capitated business, your net revenue would decrease, skewing the percentage. This approach is not recommended.

A second approach is to identify synergies from the integration or process improvement and estimate the savings. As Table 5-1 illustrates, a process of identifying where savings could occur will point to potential dollar savings.

A third method is to identify net revenues, then add in your expenses. You will often be able to predict from historical trends what your net revenues will be for the following year. Your bottom line or net income may be dictated by senior leadership. In Table 5-2, senior leadership required a net income of 10% of net revenue. Once you know your net revenues, the optimal supplies, and other costs, plug in wages to achieve a balance. Obviously, the potential change cannot affect quality negatively.

Depending on your market environment, a 2% net income may be easily attained, whereas a 5% net income may be a challenge.

A fourth approach would be to have cost per test as a goal. The intangibles that cannot be measured with a cost-per-test analysis are accuracy and service. If wages are the most expensive item and you have optimized technology and design (most have not), then service and quality may decrease to get to a lower cost per test. Continued improvement in technology can be purchased, but the savings must support those decisions. Organizations must recognize that cost reduction is not just a matter of adjusting budgets.

TABLE 5-1. *Synergy Savings*

Technical Staff	Location A FTEs	Location B FTEs	Combined	After synergy reduction	Average cost per FTE	Wages to be saved
Hematology	3	3	6	6	$30,000	0
Auto chem	2	3	5	4	$30,000	$30,000
Spec chem	2	4	6	4	$30,000	$60,000
Serology	0.5	3.5	4	1.5	$35,000	$87,500
Microbiology	3	15	18	15	$40,000	$120,000
Total savings in wages						$297,500

TABLE 5-2. *Plugging to your goal (0,000)*

Known net revenues	$10
Expenses:	
Wages	$ 4 (plug)*
Known supply costs	$ 3
Known other costs	$ 2
Net income goal	$ 1

RESULTS OF HAVING A SPECIFIC GOAL

We spent many hours discussing the laboratory's need to reduce expenses and duplication. Until we had a tangible $800,000 goal, we could not successfully address many key issues. Initially, there was an effort to delicately avoid any discussion about reducing FTEs (full-time equivalents, 40 hours worked per week). It became apparent when we started putting dollar amounts next to suggested improvements that a reduction in FTEs was necessary. Approximately 50% of the cost reduction would be related to FTE reductions. This would demand a significant process improvement if we were going to maintain our current level of quality and service.

With the specific dollar goal, the process of exploring the necessary changes started to fall into place. There were several meetings where participants argued about why something could not be done. One example was serology. The medical technologists were putting in overtime and felt that the serology process was already maximized. We eventually moved all serology from the hospital to the core laboratory, streamlined the processes, and reduced 3.5 FTEs to 1.5 FTEs. There was no reduction in service but non-value-added steps were eliminated. One step that had been a part of the previous process was to correlate any *coccidioidomycosis* serological testing with previous results. It was agreed that this was the responsibility of the clinician and was readily available in the patient's office chart. An additional time-consuming step was verifying all hospital HIV consent forms. In the revised process, this was discussed with nursing, and the consent became the responsibility of the nursing units. These were some of the changes that resulted in significant time and dollars saved.

The status quo was no longer acceptable. Having a specific dollar goal that everyone knew gave us a reality check. A sensitive issue and common debate was that quality would suffer. Quality and cost generally track each other. In other words, poor quality resulting from such issues as repeat testing, dealing with complaints, and potential negative impact on patient care cost the system in many ways. We had to make sure that the new processes we created did not negatively affect quality. We did this by constant monitoring, using multiple customer surveys as well as a published phone number specifically for problems. Less repeat testing and early identification of customer concerns improved quality and was more cost-effective.

Because of the short time allotted for completion of our integration (less than a year), we could not avoid layoffs. Discussions of the number of positions should be based on good financial data and should be communicated in a timely fashion to avoid rumors, which can be more devastating than the truth. In today's environment there are no job guarantees. The most common question was, "Am I going to have a job?" The answer was, "We don't know."

UNITS OF PRODUCTION (UNITS OF SERVICE, VOLUME OF WORK)

Whether it is called *units of service*, *units of production*, *transactions*, *billing units*, or *requisitions*, there needs to be a common and consistent way to compare volume of work. We were fortunate that we had a relatively good comparison of volume between the two sites (hospital and reference lab) in our first integration. Whether you are going through a merger or not, it is worthwhile to track units of production as an internal benchmark. The computer systems at each location can influence the ease of developing valid comparisons. We download all tests into an SAS database program daily. SAS is an over-the-counter software program that is excellent for manipulating large data files. This is not a product that is easily taught or used by the average person. In our lab one individual is responsible for the database. We use SAS because of its ability to manipulate large data files quickly and its flexibility in producing both statistical and financial information, such as monthly and yearly comparisons and market information. (The information can be compressed, so disk space is not an issue.)

Using this program, we manipulate the data to meet specified criteria, such as exploding a chemistry profile into many tests, counting a chemistry profile as one test, or counting STAT requests separately. A database program such as SAS provides the ability to manipulate data quickly, offering better storage and retrieval than most turnkey systems. Table 5-3 gives some examples of valuable information applicable to most projects. Last month and year-to-date should be used for statistical trending. These data can be used to internally benchmark to the previous year.

Information such as ordering physician, collection site, referral physician, test volume, and net revenue is also available. (Third-party payers frequently want information of this type.) Using the SAS database, you could obtain the volume of CBCs from Doctors Jones, Smith, Sonders, and Johnson from a specific time period as a percent of total volume, sorted by the collection sites. Again, the negative side of using a database system such as SAS is that you need an experienced programmer. It is not a turnkey system.

Information on larger turnkey laboratory information systems (LIS) is moved periodically to an external disk or tape. Access to past information is more difficult to retrieve compared with a file in SAS. Most LIS systems are not as flexible with regard to data management, and valuable LIS system resources may be slowed down when running a query.

Seasonal trends can influence decisions negatively if adequate samples are not obtained. In warmer climates, such as Arizona, population and business increase in the winter. To avoid misleading trends keep multiple years of data.

TABLE 5-3. *Monthly volume and statistic report (July 1996)*

Test	Volume per month	Percent of total	YTD volume	Percent of total
CBC	385	20.69	2,785	20.40
Platelet	256	13.76	1,795	13.15
Testosterone	12	0.64	102	0.75
Urinalysis	186	9.99	1,255	9.19
TSH	996	53.52	7,522	55.11
T3 (Free)	26	1.40	190	1.39
Total	1,861		13,649	

CRITERIA FOR SELECTING A GOOD DATA MANAGEMENT SYSTEM

Fast and flexible.
PC based.
Able to download to other software.
Able to sort, query, and save large amounts of data.

Both computer and financial planning/analyst can assist in identifying a system that will meet your needs.

For the merger we wanted to review comparative data for the hospital and the core lab. We decided to group like departments and processes to test the validity of our financial information. The hospital had separate departments for hematology, chemistry, urinalysis, and coagulation. The commercial laboratory had one department, and medical technologists worked in most technical areas of the laboratory. The data for the hospital showed accurate costs for FTEs per section. At the core laboratory, we could only speculate on FTEs per section based on volume and duration of time to perform tests. We combined the departments in the hospital into one department for purposes of comparison.

It is very important to choose a standard that is user-friendly and works for multiple projects. We use the Medicare standard, with some minor adjustments, for identifying units. The following are some guidelines we used when choosing a method for identifying units of service.

1. *A standard that won't frequently change.* Using a consistent standard provides ongoing comparisons for future projects as well as internal and external benchmarking.

   Your next project may require you to provide information similar to a past project. If your standard for identifying volume has not changed, you will be able to use prior information. Using a consistent standard provides ongoing comparisons for the future.

2. *A standard that changes for everyone.* In today's changing environment, where laboratories are either merging, buying, or partnering, you need to make sure that your standard is universally accepted. The Medicare standard for identifying tests does change, but the changes are the same for everyone across the board.

3. *A standard that can be used for multiple projects.* Billing should have a strong tie to the units of service, simplifying data management in such areas as market or workload analysis. For example, the standard used in billing may not apply to courier analysis. Using one standard across your laboratory can result in duplicate analysis. Multiple standards could make it difficult comparing areas or looking for trends. Select one standard, when possible, that can be used for multiple projects.

4. *A standard that is easily reproducible.* The way Medicare counts is consistent throughout the United States and is easily reproducible. You may develop a model or tool, use it, and then scrap it because it does not provide the information you want for the next project. Medicare changes nationwide, is easily benchmarked, and generally works regardless of the project.

   Some choose a standard designed to produce a positive image for the laboratory. For example, counting STAT orders or blood products may be needed for statistical purposes, but counting them as a unit of work or a test is questionable. When comparing with another laboratory that uses the Medicare standard, higher volumes created using a different standard could be viewed as misleading and could affect credibility.

COST DEFINITIONS

Full Costs

Full costs include space, utilities, supplies, administrative support, and so on (see Table 5-4). Many question the use of full costs, because some, such as facility expenses, are thought to be fixed and therefore do not matter. They argue that no matter how many tests you do, the facility costs stay the same. If your analysis is used to identify sites to perform tests, a more expensive site would affect your decision. You will not identify this with marginal costing where you only look at the expense to produce one more test. Determining full costs is absolutely necessary in mergers where decisions such as testing sites are involved.

Overhead allocation is significant in full-cost analysis. The accounting department may place a portion of the non-revenue-generating functions, such as transportation or administration, into one overhead allocation account that is then charged to the revenue-generating departments such as pharmacy or laboratory. If you are being charged an overhead allocation expense, ask the following questions: "Is the expense valid?" "Without being able to determine your own make-or-buy decisions on services such as printing, laundry, transportation, laboratory information services (LIS), and so on, how do you know if costs are fairly allocated?" You are not in control of areas where you could po-

TABLE 5-4. *Full cost comparison*

	1997 Partner 1 per BU	1997 Partner 2 per BU	1997 Partner 3 per BU	Combined All partners per BU
SW&B	$ — 0.00	$ — 0.00	$ — 0.00	— 0.00
Salary and wages	$ — 0.00	$ — 0.00	$ — 0.00	— 0.00
Benefits	$ — 0.00	$ — 0.00	$ — 0.00	— 0.00
Op supplies	— 0.00	— 0.00	— 0.00	— 0.00
Other	— 0.00	— 0.00	— 0.00	— 0.00
Other purchasing	— 0.00	— 0.00	— 0.00	— 0.00
Indirect (allocation)	— 0.00	— 0.00	— 0.00	— 0.00
Courier expenses	— 0.00	— 0.00	— 0.00	— 0.00
Travel and ent	— 0.00	— 0.00	— 0.00	— 0.00
Send-out testing	— 0.00	— 0.00	— 0.00	— 0.00
Consulting	— 0.00	— 0.00	— 0.00	— 0.00
Corp. services	— 0.00	— 0.00	— 0.00	— 0.00
Rent/utilities	— 0.00	— 0.00	— 0.00	— 0.00
Repair/maint. facil.	— 0.00	0.00	0.00	— 0.00
Billing expenses	— 0.00	— 0.00	— 0.00	— 0.00
Telecommunications	— 0.00	— 0.00	— 0.00	— 0.00
Insurance	— 0.00	— 0.00	— 0.00	— 0.00
Miscellaneous	— 0.00	— 0.00	— 0.00	— 0.00
Misc taxes	— 0.00	— 0.00	— 0.00	— 0.00
Depreciation & amortization	— 0.00	— 0.00	— 0.00	— 0.00
Bad debt	— 0.00	— 0.00	— 0.00	— 0.00
Billing units (BU)	1.0	1.0	1.0	3.0
Total expenses	—	—	—	—
Expense per BU	0.00	0.00	0.00	0.00

tentially save money. Consolidating efforts such as printing services may reduce overall expenses for your hospital or system but may negatively affect the lab. A more valid overhead allocation would be based on usage of service. An overhead allocation related to merely assigning a percent of the overhead is an easy way for accounting to do its job but does not accurately reflect your cost and therefore your bottom line. These overhead allocations are sometimes based on such factors as number of employees, square footage, and so on, which do not reflect usage.

During our integration, we discovered that the hospital cost per test was not fully loaded with all costs. The hospital cost per test included only direct costs such as salaries and operating supplies. It did not include facilities and employee benefits. The commercial laboratory was fully loaded with all costs. We performed an analysis that included those expenses that gave us a fair comparison.

Marginal Costs

Marginal costing is the cost to produce one additional test and should not be used when looking for synergies or deciding on testing sites. For example, if a doctor wanted to send one additional test, the cost of expenses, such as courier services, is already included and would not change. Pricing on the margin may allow you to acquire additional business and spread your fixed expenses over more volume. This is how volume discounting is justified for reference labs. Marginal costing should not be used when developing synergies.

Another common approach to determine test cost is to identify wages, supplies, and equipment to produce a single test. This method is time-consuming and does not take into account such items as quality control, maintenance, or other overhead allocations. This approach is sometimes used to price on the margin. Again, full cost, which includes all costs of the laboratory, is the most accurate method to identify where synergies may occur.

Direct Costs

Direct costs include expenses such as wages, benefits, supplies, reagents, controls, calibrators, and instruments. This category includes all costs directly associated with test production in a department.

Indirect Costs

Indirect costs include areas such as courier expenses, billing, and administrative expenses. Indirect costs are those expenses not directly related to the production of test results.

Many hospitals do not list indirect costs in the departmental expense reports. However, it is beneficial to include them in a comparison to see if all sites are charged equally. It is hard to determine the indirect costs if they are allocated. For example, our inpatient hospital laboratory billing is accomplished through the hospital billing function. Laboratory participation on this billing is almost nonexistent. The core laboratory had a separate billing function that allowed it to know the exact cost of billing per unit of service. In our merger we decided not to include the cost of billing because it was not relevant to the outcome and there was minimal opportunity for synergy.

Fixed Costs

Fixed costs do not or cannot change with volume. A 24-hour-a-day, 7-day-a-week operation must staff at least one technologist regardless of volume, and this is a fixed expense. In a team-oriented environment, having a technologist perform other tasks such as purchasing, stocking, typing, or even sweeping the floors can offset fixed expense. Our laboratory structure needs to transport specimens from the hospital laboratory to the commercial laboratory 24 hours a day, 7 days a week. Because there is not a constant need for the courier on the night shift, the courier stocks and orders supplies at slow times. Fixed costs, such as the price of an instrument, either fully goes away or fully stays with any process change.

Variable Costs

Variable costs can and do change with volume. The best examples of variable costs are consumable supplies and salary and wages of hourly production staff. Volume changes impact supplies and staffing. Flexible staffing, which is not always well accepted, is a key factor in controlling variable costs.

Many hospitals in warm resort areas, such as Arizona, have seasonal volume changes, when the winter population increases approximately 10%. Flexible staffing is a key factor in controlling variable costs.

Identification of Potential Synergy

Synergy is the benefit derived from combining activities. To develop synergy, you must identify fixed and variable costs, specific lab overhead allocation expenses, and units of production. If the productivity standard for one technologist is 25,000 tests per year but each testing site performs only 20,000 tests per year, and a technologist must be at each site 8 hours per day to perform these tests, then the technologist would not be at maximum efficiency. If you combined this operation (40,000 tests) and eliminated a site, then you could meet the 8-hour-per-day criterion and have 1.6 technologists on staff (40,000/25,000). At an annual salary of $35,000, this represents a $14,000 savings. Synergy will reduce duplicated fixed expenses such as equipment and service contracts. We moved routine testing to the outside commercial laboratory to take advantage of excess instrument capacity and perform more batch testing, which requires fewer controls and less technical time.

To identify synergies of integration, we used spreadsheets that developed a proforma based on volume and expense changes. This spreadsheet has multiple folders linked to a final 5-year proforma based on future assumptions such as volume changes and capital requirements. The first year of the proforma would be before merging or process improvement. Table 5-5 gives an example of this program.

It is important that you identify all aspects of synergy. For example, the cost of moving instruments and any severance expenses should be included. Projections based on the best available data are used to predict the success of a venture.

Each project should be justified using a 5-year cash flow and net present value. A 5-year cash flow allows you to see the entire cash outlays and inflows over the life of the project, or a reasonable time frame. We use a 5-year cash flow for all projects, whether they be capital acquisitions, leases, new businesses, or position justifications. A 5-year

TABLE 5-5. *Potential savings*

Function	1997 Part-ner 1 FTE	1997 Part-ner 1 SWB$	1997 Part-ner 2 FTE	1997 Part-ner 2 SWB$	1997 Part-ner 3 FTE	1997 Part-ner 3 SWB$	1997 Com-bined FTES	Consolidated Combined SWB$	Consolidated Combined FTE	SWB$
Courier	0	$0	0	$0	0	$0	0	$0	0	$0
Phleb—hospital	0	$0	0	$0	0	$0	0	$0	0	$0
Phleb—collection sites	0	$0	0	$0	0	$0	0	$0	0	$0
Sales mgr	0	$0	0	$0	0	$0	0	$0	0	$0
Field service reps	0	$0	0	$0	0	$0	0	$0	0	$0
Specimen proc/core	0	$0	0	$0	0	$0	0	$0	0	$0
Specimen proc/hospital	0	$0	0	$0	0	$0	0	$0	0	$0
Finance/Acctg	0	$0	0	$0	0	$0	0	$0	0	$0
Sect/clerical support	0	$0	0	$0	0	$0	0	$0	0	$0
Administration	0	$0	0	$0	0	$0	0	$0	0	$0
Billing	0	$0	0	$0	0	$0	0	$0	0	$0
Billing/data ent.	0	$0	0	$0	0	$0	0	$0	0	$0
Payroll	0	$0	0	$0	0	$0	0	$0	0	$0
A/P	0	$0	0	$0	0	$0	0	$0	0	$0
HR	0	$0	0	$0	0	$0	0	$0	0	$0
Directors	0	$0	0	$0	0	$0	0	$0	0	$0
Managers	0	$0	0	$0	0	$0	0	$0	0	$0
QA/QC	0	$0	0	$0	0	$0	0	$0	0	$0
Cytology	0	$0	0	$0	0	$0	0	$0	0	$0
Histology	0	$0	0	$0	0	$0	0	$0	0	$0
Stat labs	0	$0	0	$0	0	$0	0	$0	0	$0
Core lab	0	$0	0	$0	0	$0	0	$0	0	$0
Ancillary testing	0	$0	0	$0	0	$0	0	$0	0	$0
Microbiology	0	$0	0	$0	0	$0	0	$0	0	$0
Serology/immunology	0	$0	0	$0	0	$0	0	$0	0	$0
Toxicology	0	$0	0	$0	0	$0	0	$0	0	$0
Blood bank	0	$0	0	$0	0	$0	0	$0	0	$0
Other	0	$0	0	$0	0	$0	0	$0	0	$0
Veterinary	0	$0	0	$0	0	$0	0	$0	0	$0
Pathology	0	$0	0	$0	0	$0	0	$0	0	$0
Clinics	0	$0	0	$0	0	$0	0	$0	0	$0
Client services	0	$0	0	$0	0	$0	0	$0	0	$0
Materials management	0	$0	0	$0	0	$0	0	$0	0	$0
Information services	0	$0	0	$0	0	$0	0	$0	0	$0
Grand total	*0*	*$0*	*0*	*$0*	*0*	*$0*	*0*	*$0*	*0*	*$0*

cash flow lets you see the financial impact of the project. Table 5-6 is an example of a 5-year cash flow for identifying the best option for acquiring a new instrument.

Allocating Indirect Costs

Most commercial laboratories have responsibility for and can track full costs of doing business, whereas hospital laboratories have overhead allocations based on indicators such as FTEs or space. Table 5-7 shows a typical hospital allocation schedule.

We decided to include only those expenses that were necessary. We did not compare the costs of utilities because their inclusion would only shift rather than reduce costs for the organization. We did include the cost of in-house maintenance on equipment. The hospital had this expense as an overhead allocation, whereas the commercial laboratory had this expense detailed on its monthly expense report. Adjusting for these expense differences brought more clarity to areas that would see the biggest dollar improvement. Many would argue that looking at allocated expenses is a waste of time. However, the ability to compare an in-house allocation of an expense with a similar expense purchased

TABLE 5-6. *Five year cash flow*

Option 1:	Purchase option					
	Year 1	Year 2	Year 3	Year 4	Year 5	Total
Outlay	$200,000	$0	$0	$0	$0	$200,000
NPV @ 10.5%	$17,391					
Option 2:	60-month FMV lease with buyout at year 2					
	Year 1	Year 2	Year 3	Year 4	Year 5	
Outlay	$48,168	$168,654	$0	$0	$0	$216,822
NPV @ 10.5%	$5,464					
OR	60-month FMV lease					
	Year 1	Year 2	Year 3	Year 4	Year 5	
Outlay	$48,168	$48,168	$48,168	$48,168	$48,168	$240,840
NPV @ 10.5%	$4,587					
Option 3:	60-month FMV lease with 6 months deferred payments and buyout at year 2					
	Year 1	Year 2	Year 3	Year 4	Year 5	
Outlay	$27,426	$191,130	$0	$0	$0	$218,556
NPV @ 10.5%	$3,830					
Option 4:	Tiered rental with optional purchase at 12 months					
	Year 1	Year 2	Year 3	Year 4	Year 5	
Outlay	$14,004	$205,104	$0	$0	$0	$219,108
NPV @ 10.5%	$2,769					
OR						
	Year 1	Year 2	Year 3	Year 4	Year 5	
Outlay	$14,004	$59,304	$59,304	$59,304	$59,304	$251,220
NPV @ 10.5%	$1,709					

NPV = net present value; FMV = fair market value. The net present value takes into account all the variables and allows you to see the actual cost or profit of the project in today's dollars.

from an outside source may give you a competitive edge. If you include allocated expenses in a merged laboratory expense proforma, then after you integrate, the expenses are still present with the hospital and need to be accounted for more accurately. Including all overhead allocation in your synergy analysis may give you a skewed savings. Some of the expenses, left with the hospital, are not a real savings unless the system treats them as variable costs. Real savings are those eliminated, not just moved elsewhere.

Units of Production

We download all information into a data base (SAS) and count units using the Medicare standards. We use these units of production to look at cost per unit of service.

TABLE 5-7. *Department allocation for the laboratory*

Department	Allocation factor	Total dollars	Department allocation
Linen and laundry	FTEs	$1,300,000	$169,000
Building maintenance	Square Ft	$5,000,000	$1,000,000
Administration	Expense $	$2,150,000	$129,000
Security	FTEs	$566,000	$73,580
Electric	Square Ft	$240,000	$48,000
Waste disposal	Square Ft	$56,000	$11,200
Print shop	Expense $	$1,800,000	$108,000
Cafeteria	FTEs	$25,060	$3,258
Risk management	Potential Liab	$6,532,000	$1,502,360
Financial services	Expense $	$256,000	$15,360
Total allocated dollars		**$17,925,060**	**$3,059,758**

This helps to identify where inefficiencies may occur. Looking at cost per unit of service helps us understand which areas of the laboratory are costing more than they should, based on internal or external benchmarking, highlighting areas for improvement.

APPROPRIATE COSTING METHOD FOR ANALYSIS

Departmental Costing

Departmental costing identifies full costs and billing units associated with a single department. A department could be a single chemistry profile instrument or a grouping of many instruments and processes. This method of costing is easy to maintain and can be very accurate because all costs are identified. You can separate these costs using departmental expense reports and volume information downloads. Departmental costing is an excellent method to use for the entire laboratory because of ease of maintenance, accuracy, and inclusion of all costs associated with producing a test. It is the best method for identifying synergy because it is detailed enough to identify where overlap, duplication, and inefficiencies occur. It is a simple method that expedites the costing process. There are many ways to do a departmental allocation. Simply identify the time spent and the supplies and equipment used; then match units to those costs. We now allocate units and expenses to areas such as special chemistry and immunology. By doing this, we can analyze departmental changes.

Full Cost

The full cost refers to all costs incurred by the laboratory. This approach is easy to maintain, but it is not best to price to market. Costs such as the courier between the core lab and the hospital would be missed if departmental or marginal costs are used. For that reason, full cost is the preferred method when looking at synergies.

NEED FOR VALID COMPARISONS OF UNITS OF SERVICE

It is common to use Medicare standards, even though some tests are not included under the Medicare accounting systems. Examples of tests that are not included would be the number of blocks in histology or timed test orders (STATs or rapid turnaround tests). Actually, counting blocks may be more accurate in determining workload in histology, but it is not the accepted standard for billing. Counting chemistry profiles consistently is a common area of concern. Chemistry profiles or organ profiles may be counted as one test or many. Profiles are a good example of why a standard such as Medicare should be used. Stratification of your data may be necessary, depending on your project. For example, in phlebotomy more effort is required for a STAT. The same applies to surgical pathology charges for complicated versus simple cases. Other details to look at are repeats, calibrations, and so on. The key is to ensure that the comparisons are fair and valid.

Getting too microscopic or detailed in your analysis can be a problem. We spent many hours identifying the cost of high-volume tests, marginal costing, and so on. In retrospect, our time could have been better spent identifying the costs of specific areas such as hematology (departmental costing). We knew the total number of tests and expenses by department. Once you know the costs per unit of service, compare them from one department to another; then review extreme variants and look for explanations of the differences.

ABC Analysis

ABC analysis is usually used in an inventory control process, but we found it very useful in identifying the location in which a test should be performed (e.g., hospital versus an outside laboratory). An A represents a critical test that cannot be moved; a B represents less critical tests that could be moved; and a C stands for routine tests where turnaround time allows performance at a central location. For example, a partial thromboplastin time (PTT) is generally urgent and should be done on site. This test would have an A rating. Basic chemistries are usually routine, with the exception of those from the Emergency Department, which are almost always urgent because of the nature of the visit. Routine tests would be given a C rating. Vancomycin levels are an example of a B test. They are ordered infrequently, require a turnaround time of 2 hours, and could be done at a remote location if you could meet the time requirements. Those tests that are only set up once a day or a few times each week are routine with rare exceptions and would be C items that are easily moved.

ABC analysis generally takes precedence over financial analysis. Patients' needs are a priority in dictating location of testing. In any merger this should be your first analysis in determining if you can move tests.

Standardization

Standardization is the process of using the same instrumentation and supplies for each location, thus reducing the number of vendors and decreasing expenses due to volume discounts. Before integration, the hospital laboratory (chemistry, hematology, urinalysis, and coagulation) had 43 different vendors and an average supply cost per billing unit of $2.01. The core laboratory, for the same departments, had 25 vendors and a supply cost per billing unit of $1.65. After integration the combined laboratory, for the same departments, had a total of 30 vendors and an average cost of $1.42. A lack of coordination among departments resulted in ordering the same items from different vendors. Standardization reduced the total number of vendors as well as ordering and accounting time. The cost to produce a purchase order has been estimated at $50 to $500. The standardization of products and vendors is significant in decreasing expenses.

Vendors in most cases are not interested in cherry picking or line-item bidding on your business. They would rather be "partners." This process essentially guarantees the vendor the opportunity to have a more fixed percentage of your business. A win/win vendor relationship can be both financially and technically positive when you are seen as a preferred customer.

ROLE OF THE COMPUTER IN PURCHASING

A computer system for the materials management process should include linkages between purchasing, accounts payable, and the general ledger. This allows for automatic audit trails. In our system an item is assigned a purchase order and each item is specific to a department and account number. Because the purchasing function is linked to the general ledger, the appropriate department is charged for the expense immediately, thus avoiding input errors. An invoice cannot be paid unless the purchase order has a receiving document input into the computer and the price on the invoice matches that on the purchase order. Thus, erroneous prices and amounts are automatically flagged. Previously, reentering invoices required a full-time employee who distributed items first into the store room and then, as they were needed, out of the store room to each department. The trail of supplies required manual input of each requested item in the computer. This process was time-consuming, offered more opportunity for mistakes, and did not add value.

MONITORING COSTS

Conduct Frequent Reviews

If you have used the tools illustrated in this chapter, it is easy to compare your performance with projected budgets. Weekly, we have a department supervisor give a financial presentation to the management team. We keep the format the same for each department and assist in preparing control charts of the performance from the perspectives of dollar variance and per-billing-unit variance. We monitor total cost, cost per billing unit (Medicare-defined units), departmental costs, and departmental cost per billing unit. Financial monitoring should be performed at least monthly. You should be able to review departmental information at any time. It is important as departmental supervisors to be a part of the preparation and presentation of this report. It results in greater knowledge of finance and more involvement once the information is accessible and known.

Continually Reevaluate Processes

We evaluated our reference laboratory pricing and identified those tests that might be performed cost-effectively in-house.

We evaluated all service contracts and identified those that could be self-insured (parts and labor paid for on an as-needed basis), limited, or unlimited requiring 24-hour-per-day, 7-day-a-week coverage, thereby finding areas where savings were possible.

Remember to review cost per test periodically and compare this cost with outsourcing when service would not be negatively affected. Be sure to look at the full costs of these tests, including space for testing, time for regulatory issues, and storage of supplies. The data must identify where there are variable costs, as well as fixed costs, with potential savings.

Bring Everything Back to a Per-Unit-of-Service Basis

We look at all costs on a per unit of service basis. The primary reason for using cost per unit of service rather than cost variance is to identify whether an increase or decrease in cost is due to volume changes or inefficiencies. An increase in volume may cause a related increase in departmental costs, even though your processes may be more efficient. We need to identify whether the variance is from volume or from cost per test. The formula to do this is relatively simple (Table 5-8).

We have departmental and subdepartmental reports that illustrate 24-month actual expenses and 24-month budget averages for the year and per billing unit. This report is used by all managers and supervisors to monitor activity for future budgeting, including justifications of positions and equipment.

We monitor expense and revenue categories, providing 15 months of data in each category. We can compare the current year with the last 3 years and see if each category is

TABLE 5-8. *Identifying source of variance*

Month's budgeted volume	185,000
Month's actual volume	188,000
Month's actual supply expense	289,000
Actual cost per billing unit	1.537
Month's budgeted supply expense	256,000
Budgeted cost per billing unit	1.384

Calculation:
  $33,000 variance in cost of supplies for the month (289,000 − 256,000)
  Variance attributed to volume = 188,000 − 185,000 = 3,000 × $1.384 = $4,200
  Variance attributed to cost = $1.54 − $1.38 = $.153 × 188,000 = $28,800

within statistical control. Using statistical process control and determining when units or costs fall outside control limits help determine when processes need to be evaluated and changes may need to be made. For example, if wage expense over the last 12-month period has an upper control limit of $9.80 per unit of service and the lower control limit is $7.68 per unit, then any month within these limits would be considered in control. If one month is higher than the last, this would be considered normal variation. If a month fell outside of the control limit, then we would look for special causes or trends related to this variation. This database provides helpful information when we want to benchmark our operation.

CONCLUSION

The impact that integration of laboratory services has on a health system's bottom line can be considerable. However, using the appropriate tools and analysis is key to identifying which savings are real and which are not. The guidelines illustrated in this chapter will help you select the appropriate tools for financial analysis.

We recently were involved with a project where we used the tools described. We quickly obtained consensus from all parties regarding our proforma and synergy analysis because it was based on logical analysis and assumptions. The assumptions were based on rational processes such as counting tests, using Medicare units, and only included those allocation expenses that would change with the project.

Using the appropriate financial tools for cost analysis is key, not only for mergers, but for day-to-day analysis and knowing your business potential. We have tried to emphasize which methods of analysis are valid in particular situations. We have also discussed shortcomings of each method of examination. Understanding financial analysis is crucial to making decisions that impact the bottom line and can impact survival. Health care is in a financial crisis, and we can ill afford to make uninformed financial decisions that affect the bottom line negatively.

6

Appropriate Utilization

Paul Bozzo

Health care costs are rising more rapidly than the cost of inflation, and the number of lab tests has increased dramatically, more than doubling since their automation in the early 1950s. Lab tests account for a significant part of the patient billing. Previously, neither patients, nor physicians had an economic incentive to restrict the number of tests ordered, because they were paid without question by the insurance company (1). The higher cost of medical care has resulted in unavailability of care for some, lower quality for others, and anxiety among physicians (2). Reimbursement for health care has been curtailed, resulting in a need to reduce costs while maintaining quality.

Approximately 80% of clinical decisions are made by physicians, including most decisions on diagnostic testing (3). There were approximately 5 billion lab tests in 1990, accounting for 5% to 7% of the health care budget (4,5). Because most labs are computerized, it is easy to obtain laboratory data related to costs and thus potential loss of income or savings for both health care providers and regulatory agencies wanting to project fairly accurate budget cuts related to reimbursement.

Appropriateness of testing refers to testing when it is clinically indicated. The phrase *clinically indicated* implies utilization standards, but patients may not fit into these standard categories. Thus it is reasonable for compliance with indications for testing to vary. Monitoring has focused on excessive testing. Theoretically, situations should also be monitored to identify tests that were not performed when they should have been. It is more difficult to review clinical symptoms and findings from the history and physical examination than to compile readily accessible test results. To review missed indications for a urinary tract culture, such as urinary frequency and pain with urination, would require time-consuming manual review of the medical record, a prospective study of patient symptoms, or computerized scanning of electronic medical records, which generally is impossible.

As we search for ways to cut costs in the laboratory, the first reaction is to work harder and improve our processes. This helps, but significant cost reduction will occur when we reduce the number of inappropriate diagnostic procedures. The savings may be not in the laboratory but in the unwarranted clinical assessment of false-positive results (6). This may be many times higher than the cost of repeat testing. Sometimes we fail to look at the potential indirect costs of a false positive, which includes the contacting of the patient, response to their concerns, return visit, additional laboratory tests, other diagnostic procedures, cancellation of surgery, emergency room visits, or even admission to a hospital. In actuality costs in the laboratory will not decrease parallel to the reduced volume. In one study a 10% reduction in utilization reduced the laboratory's costs by less than 2%, and a 50% reduction would have saved no more than 20% of costs (7). Fixed costs—such as those for equipment, the structure, and billing—may stay the same or vary little as a result of volume. If you are leasing equipment based on test volume, cost of variables such as reagents could actually increase. This is less true with larger labs, which have volumes that allow lower pricing of reagents and equipment.

Changing ordering patterns requires a change in behavior which potentially occurs when physicians envision a potential gain. The old adage, "What's in it for me?" applies to medicine. There should be some positive gain to the physician and/or his patient. We want to eliminate non-value-added testing; this would be positive for both the patient and the doctor. Providing data to prove that the change is positive may be easier said than done, but it is critical to promoting change. Time saved not pursuing misleading results is a positive for both the clinician and patient. The difficulty lies in the fact that the change must occur before comparative data can be collected. If the changes suggested do not result in more effective and more efficient care, they should be rejected. (The term *effective* in this context refers to doing the right thing; *efficient* refers to doing it right. Being efficient in test performance is not worth much if the test is not indicated.)

In the present environment the number of hassle factors (increased paperwork, more documentation to utilize specialists, productivity standards) and the amount of administrative control have increased dramatically. Doctors feel they're losing control of their ability to care for their patients; therefore they frequently resist change. Keeping this in mind, it is reasonable to examine why clinicians order a lab test. Modern criteria for a lab test should be whether or not it provides new, useful information. In other words, the result of testing must translate into changes in therapy or diagnosis, or represent a prognostic indicator. Physicians also order laboratory tests to screen healthy individuals, hoping to detect occult disease; to confirm or reject clinical impressions; to monitor treatment; to provide prognosis; to conduct research; to defend against possible legal liability; and to conform to patients' demands. Not all these reasons are acceptable. Appropriate ordering of tests can save a clinician's time and result in improved care. We shall discuss this later in more detail.

MALPRACTICE AS A REASON FOR ORDERING TESTS

Savings that could result from curbing defensive medicine are estimated at $7 to $8 billion per year. A nationally syndicated publication states, "Doctors perform millions of useless procedures at an annual cost estimated at $20 billion." These figures seem exaggerated but not necessarily to the public, especially when the source is the former Secretary of Health, Education, and Welfare of the United States (8). One study found that 80% of 1,000 Americans surveyed believed doctors ordered unnecessary tests to avoid being sued (9). Unfortunately, in our present medical–legal climate, we continue to do a significant number of laboratory tests, theoretically to eliminate the legal liability. This continues despite literature that shows unnecessary testing increases, not decreases, the medical–legal risk (10). There is no way to validly estimate the financial impact of testing done for medical–legal reasons. Surveys show that 75% to 98% of physicians practice defensive medicine. One of the most common practices adopted is increased diagnostic testing (11–13). We must convince clinicians that the additional testing does not prevent malpractice lawsuits and, in fact, may increase them, if abnormal results, no matter how slight, are not followed up. Malpractice claims are difficult, if not impossible, to represent if a test is not performed when there are no related symptoms. On the other hand, not following up on an abnormal test results is a bonanza for the plaintiff's lawyer when a serious illness is discovered.

SCREENING TESTS

Some argue that testing should only be ordered as a result of signs and symptoms of disease. Should screening of nonsymptomatic patients be limited to a few tests with a significant yield of abnormal results? The strongest argument for wellness screening is early intervention, which would avoid costly treatment. Those opposed to mass screening point to the low sensitivity and cost of following up on false positives. Ignoring borderline abnormal lab tests, which may appear to represent failure to recognize an abnormality, can come from a complex judgment involving the degree of abnormality and likelihood that further investigation will affect therapy (14). Or it may come as a result of knowing that a particular test is frequently slightly abnormal. The question remains, "Do we need to order as much testing as we are presently doing?" If we continue to order large non-symptom-related chemistry profiles, we will have more false positives than true positives. Electrolyte testing is a good example. If the patients are healthy and on no diuretics, the ratio of false positives to true positives may be as high as 20 to 1. (This was calculated based on a prevalence of 1 in 1,000 and a sensitivity and specificity of 98% for each test [15].) An example of ineffective testing would be ordering a uric acid test to exclude gout. In this situation, if there are no risk factors or symptoms, you would not treat the patient. Screening for hyperlipidemia, cervical cancer (Pap smears), and colorectal cancer (occult bloods) is well accepted. The value of other tests, including prostate and thyroid screening, continues to be debated.

Because normal reference ranges for tests are based on a Gaussian distribution curve, if one test is performed, approximately 5% of normal patients will show abnormal results (outside of two standard deviations). If you do a profile of 20 chemistry tests, statistically there is more than a 65% chance that you will have a false positive. The sensitivity of a test represents the percentage that will have a disease. We want to deal with tests that not only are sensitive but have a high specificity; that is, a high percentage of those who do not have the disease will have a negative test. The argument against mass screening is that both the specificity and sensitivity are low and not cost-effective.

Some authors have noted an increase in the number of orders when physicians are covering for large groups and they do not know all the patients. In addition, as the number of patients covered by managed care increases, patients are selecting new doctors. In both these situations, the clinicians will reexamine patients and request duplicate and new laboratory tests (16).

Appropriate testing (other than wellness screening) should confirm the clinical impression, answer a question raised by the history and physical, monitor treatment, or provide prognostic information. Research protocols constitute a unique situation.

Patient demands related to a recently read article or a commercial presentation that sparked the patient's curiosity should result in a dialogue and not a reflex test order. Recently, I talked to approximately 20 clinicians who pointed out that testing demands were dictated by society. The media promotes a test using medical experts from well-known institutions. The patients argue in a knowledgeable way that the test is indicated. At times, the media have promoted testing based on minimal confirmation of the medical literature. If the physician refuses to order the test, the patient's assumption is that cost, not the patient's needs, is the primary concern. Sound, well-based medical judgment of the patient's needs should be the deciding factor for ordering tests. We cannot recommend testing that is not cost-effective.

CHANGING PHYSICIAN BEHAVIOR

Changing behavioral patterns is difficult. Education, peer review, intense utilization review, administrative changes, penalties, and rewards have all been tried with varying degrees of success. What is required is a champion who will be tenacious, uses one-on-one educational efforts, and continues in the face of adversity. When the educational efforts that produced change are withdrawn, however, the program will likely return to baseline.

One successful method has been to recruit respected physicians of the community to champion a specific change. Another has been to recognize groups of innovative clinicians more likely to change, and to get this group to provide the initial nidus that embraces change and promotes growth. Educational efforts may be temporary; more permanent success may come from changing attitudes about cost-effective medical care.

Marketing change must focus on the benefits to the clinicians or their patients. If it is seen as cost cutting to benefit a system, which has an adversarial relationship with the physicians, it is doomed to failure.

Other techniques of changing behavior include the promise of a study. For example, publishing a directive that a certain test order will be scrutinized can result in a temporary decrease in the number of orders, but doing this without commitment to a more permanent change is unwise. Administrative techniques such as change in the request slip will result in decrease of those tests no longer published on the available requisition. This works best when accompanied by a dialogue about the tests eliminated. (See the discussion of thyroid testing in this chapter.) One example would be eliminating urinalysis and substituting urinalysis culture, if indicated. We instituted this change at one hospital and simultaneously provided data on the large number of negative cultures when the accompanying urinalysis was negative. The result was a significant, permanent drop in the number of negative cultures and an increase in the percentage of positive cultures. This change in ordering pattern remains stable after 2 years. Publishing prices (not costs) of diagnostic tests works as long as the price tag is easily visible at the time of the order. Physicians are still sensitive to price even though this applies only to a small percentage of the patient population. There is a limit to how much you can attach to the chart. Publishing the prices on a requisition slip works, if the doctor personally uses the requisition slip. This has been done many times with only temporary success; usually the number of orders returns to baseline within a few months of cessation of publishing the prices (17). An ideal way to use this process is to convince the clinician to use the computer to place orders. The monitor could automatically show the prices and any recent price change as the test is requested. The key for this, as well as timely messages, is to have the clinicians personally enter data into the computer.

Those who instigate change must use an approach that faciliates visualization of how change affects the patient's total health care experience. Some changes are possible when a discipline works in a vacuum, but significant changes require the cooperation of multiple disciplines, including support from the administration. Saving money in the laboratory is not worthwhile if the patient's length of stay is extended unnecessarily or if there is increased mortality or morbidity. The argument that the shortened turnaround time of laboratory results yields improved outcome for the patient is one of the unproven arguments for more point of care testing.

Finding variation is the initial step to developing a consensus pathway. Major factors contributing to variation in laboratory test ordering include such characteristics as how sick the patient is, the patient's ability to pay, physician training, physician proficiency, physician values, level of certainty required, and disagreement and uncertainty on policies and rules evolved from research sciences. Scientific evidence describing what is known, or knowable, and how this relates to clinical decisions is extremely important. The manner in which clinical policies are developed to guide individual patient-related decisions and the way they are disseminated can be the difference between failure and success (18). If there is significant variation from one similar situation to another, then there is room for discussion on how to reach consensus. Finding and demonstrating this is key to creating positive change. Most physicians, when it is pointed out that they are requesting more testing than is usual, typically respond, "My practice is different." In my experience, looking at average age, gender, and case mix has shown that this is not true. Examination of a large number of internal medicine practices revealed that the average ages were within a range of 1–2 years and there was little difference in the distribution of male and female patients. It is obvious that older patients require more testing. This is reflected in managed care's willingness to pay a higher capitation for patients over 65.

Changing behavior is challenging, difficult, and frustrating, but it is possible. Positive changes are possible that, when presented and dialogued using good data, will be accepted and improve the quality of health care.

Preadmission Testing

Approximately $30 billion is spent on preoperative testing. It has been estimated that 60% to 75% of this amount is unnecessary (19). There are no strict requirements for preoperative testing, and there is considerable variation in the process.

Preadmission testing eliminates unnecessary last-minute cancellation or delays of surgery. Maximum cost efficiency is achieved by ordering only those tests that are necessary for the surgery and will contribute to a better outcome. Effective selection of diagnostic procedures can contribute significant cost savings.

This process looked at variation in preadmission orders on knee and hip replacements as an opportunity for improving care and reducing cost. Whenever there is variation in a specific area that shows many common features, there is an opportunity for improvement. The causes of variation are many and can be physician or patient related. Consensus on the process can result in cost savings and improved care.

Just as variation can suggest excess testing, it can also point to insufficient testing.

A team led by Dolores Marshall, administrative leader, preadmission services, outpatient nursing services, and Tyler Kent, medical director of quality improvement for surgical services at Tucson Medical Center, studied the presurgical testing for joint procedures. Facilitation of the process was done by Kathy Tanner from our continuous process improvement group. The team had two champions and a facilitator skilled in moving through the data collection, dialogue, and decision making. Dialogue without direction is seldom useful. Commitment and skills are equally important.

The team noted variation in the individual clinician's approach to diagnostic procedures preoperatively. Physicians from the same orthopedic group had more similarities but were still different in their approaches. The process for change included education (literature), review of variation among physicians, administration (see preadmission form), and one-on-one advocacy by the physician and nurse leaders of the process. Early on, it became clear that anesthesiologists play a key role in determining the need for preoperative information. One of the anesthesiologists who was asked to participate became intimately involved with the development of the process and assumed the role of advocate.

The team also included participants from multiple areas that affected the patient. Included (either as a member of the team or as invited consultants) were orthopedic surgeons, anesthesiologists, cardiologists, pulmonologists, pathologists, radiologists, and personnel from scheduling, admitting, statistical support, blood bank, orthopedics, preadmission service, case management, and EKG (cardiac, noninvasive services).

As with any change, we recognize that physicians demand more than cost savings to proceed. The key to any success is the ability to measure improved outcome or, at a minimum, no adverse effect on outcome. The difficulty is that some outcome measurements are immediate and others are more remote. In this case, we did not anticipate an improved outcome, nor did we expect an adverse response to the proposed regimen. Adverse responses related to the changes that could be measured included cancellations, delays, return to the operating room for bleeding, postoperative bleeding, or infection. We felt that the suggested changes would result in additional worthwhile data for the clinicians, but we were more concerned with excessive testing. The SF36 form (a nationally used survey form), which is used in many institutions to measure functional outcomes, would allow for easy bench marking. Having this in place prior to this process to use as a baseline and having Chris Arslanian, who was experienced in the use and interpretation of this form, to supervise the collection of data made the process more valid and credible.

The SF36 is an extensive form designed for specific procedures such as total knee replacement. The questions address not only pain but ability to perform specific everyday activities, such as climbing stairs, spending time with friends, and taking part in sports.

We also measured 1 year's case mix data (all knee and hip replacements) on diagnostic test utilization before and after the changes were instituted. There was a significant decrease in the ordering of chemistry profiles, erythrocyte sedimentation rates, and bleeding times (Fig. 6-1). We continue to discuss the prothrombin times. This demonstrates the continuous effect of dialogue on the preoperative bleeding times utilization (Fig. 6-2).

We emphasized that the proposed recommendations were guidelines that could be varied to meet the patients' needs. Special care was taken to preserve the involvement of the primary care physician to eliminate the need for duplicate testing and to have previous

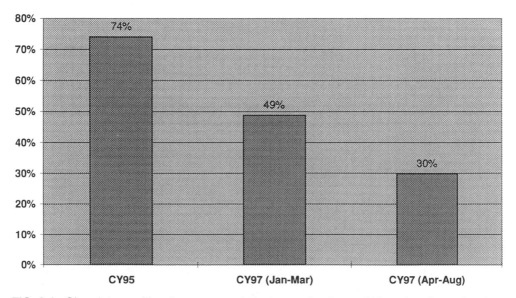

FIG. 6-1. Chemistry profiles done on preadmission testing for total hip arthroplasty showing a decreased utilization (comparison of 1995 with 1997) related to educational efforts and utilization of the new form.

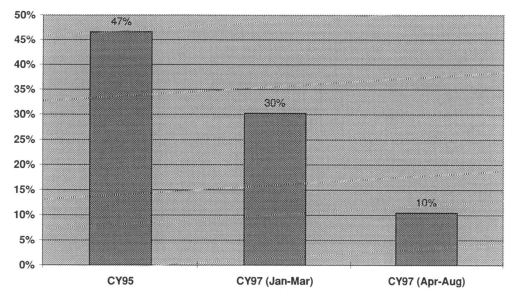

FIG. 6-2. Total bleeding times done on preadmission testing for total hip arthroplasty showing a decreased utilization (comparison of 1995 with 1997) related to educational efforts and utilization of the new form.

diagnostic data available on the chart. Our guidelines included acceptance of patient testing done in the previous 6 months.

Note how much opportunity for positive intervention would have been lost by focusing only on the orthopedic surgeon. Throughout the process we stressed that efficient and effective preoperative management still relies heavily on a thorough history and physical examination. Because of this, involvement of the primary care physician was essential. A chart of preadmission orders was not compiled without considerable dialogue. The goal was to have our preadmission form be concise, be user-friendly, and contain all the needed information. We kept saying, "Let's keep it simple." For example, the initial lists from which one line was finalized for EKG included the following items denoting clinical indications for performing an electrocardiogram preoperatively:

- Chest pain not ascribed to any etiology
- Angina or anginal equivalents
- History of congestive heart failure or its equivalent
- Diabetes
- Hypertension
- History or symptoms of dysrhythmias
- Shortness of breath
- History of myocardial infarction
- Smoking or history of smoking
- Age 50 for both men and women
- Inability to exercise without shortness of breath (SOB) or chest pain
- A need for vascular surgery.

This was reduced to EKG, cardiac symptoms, smoker, diabetes mellitus, age >50.

One goal was to eliminate lab tests that had no value for managing routine total joints. These included the following:

- Chemistry profile 16 or 20
- Complete blood count with manual differential
- Sedimentation rate
- Bleeding time
- Full coagulation profile

A study from the Mayo Clinic found abnormal values in 160 of 3,782 presurgical chemistry profiles, but only 47 (1.2%) were previously unknown. Thirty of the 160 were predictable based on the history and physical examination. No surgical procedures were delayed and no association was found between adverse outcomes and any preoperative laboratory abnormality. Because of this the Mayo Clinic no longer requires preoperative lab screening in healthy patients (20). Our approach was to exclude chemistry profiles from the requisition. We reviewed erythrocyte sedimentation rates for a month and found 34% abnormal. Many of these were ordered as screening tests. The value of a test that is abnormal in approximately 40% of the population is questionable. Sedimentation rates, bleeding times, and coagulation profiles have a low specificity. We had included a hemoglobin and hematocrit but felt that the white blood count and differential had too many variations that were nonspecific.

Coagulation Testing in the Preadmission Work-up

Bleeding times, which are frequently requested preoperatively, have such a low specificity (less than 5%) that we should question their use in patients with no bleeding history. These account for $68 million of testing per year (21). According to Doug Triplett (Ball Memorial Hospital, Muncie, Indiana, personal communication), a leading authority on coagulation, because of the low specificity and the resultant follow-up, bleeding times are the most expensive coagulation test. The bleeding time test is a poor screening test in a low-risk population (no history of bleeding disorder). The test has a low positive predictive value used as a screening test. There is considerable variation in test results because of technical variation in performing the tests. The bleeding time does not predict excessive bleeding in a patient on aspirin, a common situation.

The best preoperative screening test to predict excessive bleeding is a carefully conducted history and physical (22). Von Willebrand's disease is a common coagulopathy, and 80% of the cases are type I, which can be treated easily. Type III is rare (approximately 1 per 1 million). Types II and III are generally easily diagnosed by history and physical examination. A careful bleeding history, including questions regarding personal or family history of postpartum or mucosal-related (nose, gastrointestinal, endometrium) bleeding not related to trauma, is more significant than the laboratory testing. Medications are available to treat or prevent bleeding complications from mild von Willebrand's disease. Blood products are occasionally required with type I. This is an important disease, but it is difficult to justify standard, preoperative coagulation orders to exclude it.

A second area of concern is hemophilia. Severe and moderate deficiencies of either factor VIII or factor IX will have a history of joint, muscle, or other soft-tissue bleeds. Minor cases may have a negative history but normal coagulation testing results. Again a careful history and physical examination is the best screen. Those with significant findings will require specific factor testing. This applies to both von Willebrand's disease and hemophilia.

This was an example of an administrative change resulting in more effective care. Previously, we had a coagulation profile that included bleeding time. Just by eliminating bleeding times from the panel we were able to decrease the utilization by 13%.

The costs of coagulation testing, although small on an individual basis, are substantial because of the high frequency of testing preoperatively and false positives. Patients scheduled for tonsillectomy on antibiotics may show borderline elevations of activated partial thromboplastin times that are normal on repeat testing. Unfortunately, a frequent reflex action to any abnormal coagulation test result is a hematology consult and additional coagulation-related testing.

There are no regulatory requirements for specific preoperative testing. Testing is dictated by the patient's history and physical examination.

There are other boxes (Pre-Admission Form; see Table 6-1) to be checked that contributed significant savings. For example, "urinalysis, culture if indicated" was meant to replace one group's standard order of urinalysis and a separate order for urine cultures on a routine basis. Routine urinary cultures date back to a vague reference from about 1980 that pointed to the urinary tract as a potential source of increased infection in the operated joint. No recent references or in-house data were available to support ordering routine preoperative urine cultures. Because some groups didn't use this at all and had experienced no increased infections, this change was well accepted. Skin testing for tuberculosis could be used instead of a chest x-ray to fulfill regulatory requirements for transfer from a more costly, high-intensive-care unit to an area of low intensive care when appropriate. If skin testing for TB was not done on admission, it could delay transfer to the lower intensive-care unit.

The crucial part of the process was utilization of the preadmission form and recruitment of key staff to be champions, including surgery-scheduling personnel. Tenacity and willingness to look at the process on an ongoing basis are necessary for success.

Analysis of autologous blood usage showed that a large number of units were not being used or, if transfused, were sometimes in response to the anemia created by the donation. Autologous blood usage exhibited considerable variation. There were many discussions of standard criteria for autologous usage and the risks and costs of autologous transfusions. One proposal from pathology, based on historical data, was that primary knee replacement should have no autologous units; primary hips, one unit; secondary procedures on knees, one unit; and secondary hip revisions, two units. This was presented but not intensively pursued. Autologous blood usage was controversial and initially tabled to promote acceptance of the concept of the preadmission process.

Tyler Kent waited for a period of 3–4 months; then he continued to pursue the matter of autologous blood usage. The central themes included the following: avoidance of such usage unless the procedure usually required a transfusion; education on the present-day risks of homologous transfusion; increased use of cell saver; and dilution techniques. He presented this to groups on more than one occasion, wrote personal letters, and continued the conversations one on one. This was a champion who was respected, was a practicing physician, felt strongly that what he was doing made a contribution to patient care, and was tenacious. His method was successful and is worth reviewing.

1. Reviewed current practices graphically and displayed consistent usage to no usage by individual physicians.
2. Compared hematocrits at the time of donation with hematocrits at the time of surgery, which showed lower hematocrits (up to 15%) related to donations done too

TABLE 6-1. *Preadmission form*

Patient's name: _____ Patient's date of birth: _____/_____/_____

Home phone: (   ) _____ Work phone: (   ) _____

Anticipated date of admission: ____ / _____ / ____ Procedure date (if different): _____ / _____ / ____
Area where procedure to be performed: (CIRCLE) **ASC   MAIN OR   L&D   TOI   RAD**

Physician **MUST WRITE:**   **"ADMIT TO INPATIENT" OR "ADMIT TO OBSERVATION"**
                          _____

                          OR — (CIRCLE)   **OUTPATIENT PROCEDURE**
Diagnosis: _____ Insurance Group: _____
Code Status: (CIRCLE)   **A   B   C   D   Allergies:** _____

Procedure to be performed (consent): _____
_____

Admit physician: _____ PCP: _____

Consult physician: _____ (Specialty): _____

Case manager:_____

READMISSION ORDERS: **(   ) Check here if PCP to be contacted for prior diagnostics.**
                    i.e.—CXR within 1 yr./EKG within 6 mos./LABS with 6 wks.

H&P (   ) Dictated Confirmation#_____ (   ) Faxed   (   ) Courier

Pre-Op Office Visit: _____PAS Date: _____

BASIC DIAGNOSTICS: (PROCEDURES WITH PROSTHETICS or POTENTIAL BLOOD LOSS)
(   ) H&H   (   ) UA Culture if indicated   (   ) PPD—(SNF Admission **REQUIREMENT**)

ADDITIONAL CLINICALLY INDICATED DIAGNOSTICS: BLOOD UTILIZATION:

TEST:	**COMMON INDICATION:**	( ) T&S _____	( ) T&C _____
( ) K+	**Diuretics, Dig., Renal disease**	( ) Cell Saver	( ) Blood Bank Hold Clot
( ) Bun, Creat	**Age > 60, Renal disease**	( ) Autologous _____	
( ) Glucose	**Obese, DM**_____		
( ) PT, PTT	**Bleeding Hx, Hepatic, Anticoagulant**	*OTHER:* (please specify)	
( ) CXR	**Active disease, Recent immigrant**		
	( ) SCD's _____ ( ) TED Hose Thigh/Knee		
( ) EKG	**Cardiac symptoms, Smoker, DM, Age > 50**	( ) Prophylactic Antibiotic _____	

ANESTHESIA GROUP: _____ (   ) Additional diagnostics _____

DAY OF PROCEDURE ORDERS:

Prep: _____ Prophylactic antibiotics: _____

OTHER/SPECIAL ORDER: _____ Prophylactic anticoag: _____

Please **FAX** this requisition to Pre-Admission Services at Tucson Medical Center—324-1851, or have the patient bring it to the Pre-Admission Services Office (northeast entrance at TMC) at the time of his/her appointment. If questions, call our office at 324-1446.

SIGNATURE ORDERING PHYSICIAN: _____
TUCSON MEDICAL CENTER

close (in time) to the operative date. (Many of the autologous donations were done 3–4 days prior to surgery.)

3. Asked for the rationale behind ordering the units. Some clinicians thought that autologous transfusions were the standard of care; others cited patient request for autologous transfusions.
4. Stressed the current data demonstrating the low risks of homologous units (blood bank units) if needed, which was seldom done with primary knee replacement.
5. Presented the potential waste and asked, "How can we change this?"
6. Again raised the question, "Do we need this?" Considering that the average cell saver salvage rate for orthopedic cases was less than 200 mL of blood, the biggest savings (potentially more than $60,000 per year), would be eliminating the use of cell saver, was on primary knee procedures. Our data shows that this approach was successful.

Figure 6-3 shows significant improvement in the utilization of autologous blood.

Additional benefits of preadmission testing to patients and their families included the opportunity to ask questions about the hospitalization (such as hours of visitation), billing, insurance concerns, and discharge planning. The latter included scheduling admission to transitional services and ability to have a wheelchair at home when required. Both of these examples could delay discharge from an acute-care bed, adding costs but no real benefit to the patient. At times, instruction in physical therapy was done on the preadmission visit. This proved beneficial, because those instructed early adapted to the therapeutic procedures more rapidly, resulting in a faster response to therapy. The preadmission visit contributed to the patient's sense of the professionalism and caring attitude of our personnel. All this helped make the patient's hospitalization not only more comfortable, but more efficient and cost-effective.

This was a sound project and economically significant. Factors favoring its success were simplicity, minimum effort on the part of the caregiver, team member's participa-

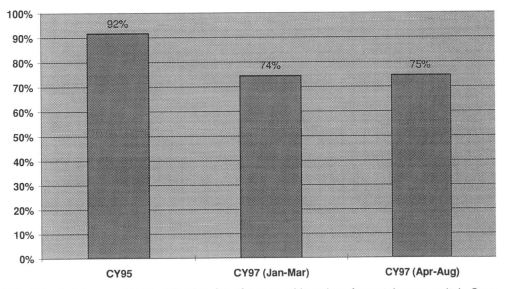

FIG. 6-3. Autologous blood utilization (% of cases with orders for autologous units). Comparison of 1995 with 1997. The improvement in utilization is primarily the result of one-on-one dialogue with the individual clinicians.

tion, and great champions. The project was a success, in large part because the behavior modification was shown to fit the clinician's paradigm shift in beliefs.

CLINICIANS BELIEFS

Previous

More test-result information
Standardized testing within groups

Now

Less testing but unique to the patient
Consensus testing criteria agreed to by multiple groups

Although designed for orthopedic joint procedures, nine months after initiating use of the form, it is being used by most of the neurosurgeons and is starting to be used in gynecology, urology, and general surgery.

Prothrombin Times/Activated Partial Thromboplastin Times (PT/APTT)

Prothrombin times/activated partial thromboplastin times (PT/APTT) are frequently ordered preoperatively by clinicians to potentially prevent bleeding during surgery. The PT measures the function of the extrinsic and common pathway of coagulation. The APTT measures the intrinsic and common pathway of coagulation. Neither test is indicated for low-risk preoperative patients.

PT/APTT testing is recommended for the following patients:

1. Clinical assessment not possible
2. Clinical evidence that suggests a bleeding disorder
3. Clinical evidence of liver disease, malnutrition, or malabsorption
4. Those for whom normal coagulation may be disrupted by the planned procedure (e.g., prostatectomy, planned use of anticoagulants, and procedures involving extracorporeal circulation)

PT/APTT testing is not recommended for low-risk patients:

LOW-RISK PATIENTS

No personal or family history of prolonged bleeding after surgery or injury
No evidence of liver disease, malabsorption, or malnutrition
Not recently on beta-lactim antibiotics
Not Ashkenazi Jew (factor XI deficiency)
Not on anticoagulants
No evidence of petechiae, ecchymosis, or hematoma

The only deficiency that PT testing detects and that APTT cannot is an isolated factor VII deficiency (one out of every 2–3 million) (23). The activated partial thromboplastin time performs poorly in predicting postoperative hemorrhage in patients without clinical suspicion of coagulopathy. Eisenberg (24) and others using PT and APTT found 13 abnormalities out of 480 patients in the low-risk group. Four were normal on repeat testing, eight went to surgery with no problems and no treatment, and one had postoperative hemorrhage, which was thought to be related to technique rather than a coagulopathy. Robbins and Rose (25) reviewed 1,000 consecutive APTT and found 143 abnormal. All had clinical findings to suggest a coagulopathy. Kaplan and associates (26) studied 154 patients without clinical indications of coagulopathy. None had an abnormal PT or APPT. Turnbull and Buck (27) reviewed 210 patients with no clinical indications of coagulopathy. Only one test was abnormal and no action was taken.

Given the data from the literature, we felt that there were too many preoperative PTs/APTTs. Many clinicians ordered PTs/APTTs on every preoperative patient. One area where we experienced slightly elevated APTTs, which were normal on repeat testing, was tonsillectomy patients who had been on antibiotics. We presented the data on three different occasions within a 3-year period at general staff meetings and in newsletters, with statistical evidence against using PTs and APTTs routinely preoperatively. There was no significant change in usage.

With no further presentations, I began to call each physician who ordered a PT/PTT as a preoperative order. This resulted in a significant decrease in the number of orders. Approximately 3 months after cessation of the calls, we were back to a baseline number of PT/APTTs. This monitor highlighted the need for tenacity and continual one-on-one education. It is well documented that we spent an excessive amount on preoperative coagulation testing. We agree with the literature that clinical assessment constitutes adequate screening in surgical and nonsurgical patients alike and that APTT and PT do not perform well in predicting intraoperative or postoperative hemorrhage (28). I plan to reinstitute calling and am presently focusing on dialogue with specific specialty groups on coagulation testing.

Chemistry Profiles/Screening Tests

With payers, including the government, considering not paying for chemistry profiles used for screening, the subject of large chemistry profiles may be of more historic than practical interest. At the time of this writing, physicians are still resistant to eliminating these profiles. A relevant goal is behavior modification to order tests specifically related to the patient's symptoms or abnormal physical findings. Chemistry profiles have become commonplace in health care, despite lack of supporting literature. In controlled studies dating back to 1976 there were no differences in length of stay, new diagnosis, or other indices of patient progress between groups having no chemistry profiles and those with them. The group that had chemistry profile testing showed more consultations, more lab tests, and a 5% higher hospital bill (29). In another study of 1,000 patients there was only one patient who might have benefited from the chemistry profile by avoiding halothane anesthesia. Many abnormals were predictable, and some were artifactual abnormalities (e.g., hemolysis related to obtaining the specimen resulting in an elevated potassium). Some abnormal results were physiologic, such as nonfasting specimens with elevated glucose or elevated results due to a decreased volume of plasma secondary to dehydration. Other findings included chemical diabetes, which would not be treated; liver disease related to excessive consumption of alcohol; and Gilberts (no treatment). There is little benefit to testing if results are predictable, known, or untreatable. In retrospect, most abnormals should have been suspected by history and physical examination (30).

Reference ranges for testing are based on distribution curves representing more than two standard deviations. Thus 5% of normal patients will have abnormal results of tests. Therefore a chemistry profile of 12 tests in an asymptomatic patient has a 46% chance of being abnormal, which most likely represents a false positive. If 20 tests are performed, there is theoretically a 65% chance of one test being abnormal. There are many slightly abnormal results that are not followed up, a potential medical–legal hazard. Large profiles continue to be popular despite the fact that an abnormal value in an asymptomatic patient is more likely to be a false positive than that in a symptomatic patient. If we used three standard deviations to define normal, we would have a smaller number of abnormals but also a decrease in the sensitivity in detecting true pathology. The cost of following up the false positives far exceeds any savings related to the lower price of a chemistry profile compared with individual tests.

Four Mayo Clinic internal medical divisions studied the value of five routine lab tests used in their outpatient setting. These included a complete blood count, lipid profile, chemistry profile, thyroid testing, and urinalysis. The lipid profile testing had the highest therapeutic yield (resultant therapeutic intervention), whereas chemistry profiles had a yield of only 2.8%. The therapeutic yield of lipid profiles was 24 times that of any of the other tests. The highest diagnostic yield in the chemistry profile was the glucose. However, treatment of type I asymptomatic diabetes mellitus is not recommended. (There is still some debate about the significance of early diagnosis of type I diabetes and the impact on the patient's medical outcome.) Overall, 11% of the individual components were abnormal, much higher than the 5% abnormals expected from a normal population. This reflects a spectrum of disease in the ambulatory population. Six percent of the abnormal tests were repeated, and 9% had additional investigative studies (31). In another study the diagnostic yield for complete blood counts was only 0.5% (32). The unresolved issue remains whether or not treating asymptomatic conditions detected by these tests is beneficial to patient care. The goal of lab test screening is to improve a patient's health by treating a newly diagnosed disease.

In the past, automated chemistry equipment performed a battery of tests on every specimen even though one or only a few tests were ordered. Today analyzers can be programmed to perform the specific tests ordered, resulting in additional savings on chemistry reagents, when specific testing rather than large panels are ordered.

Recently we lowered the price of the individual tests and eliminated chemistry profiles. We continue to offer organ profiles such as liver panels and renal panels. In related discussions, the clinicians focused on patient demands more than on patient needs. Most patients are used to having a large number of tests performed as part of their annual visit to the doctor. Societal demands are an important issue that may be overcome by third-party payers refusing to routinely compensate for large numbers of tests unrelated to findings on the history and physical examination of the patient.

Duplicate Testing

We monitored repeat chemistry profiles of hospitalized patients when all parameters were normal on the first chemistry profile. In the initial study, 19% of chemistry profiles were repeated that initially had been normal. Letters of inquiry were sent regarding the rationale for the second profile. If there was no response to the letter, I called the ordering physician. The most common cause for repeating a test was an order by a second physician who did not know of the initial order or results. In a follow-up study 10% of normals were repeated. Thus there was improvement, but duplication still remained an issue.

If the physician had to look at a computer monitor and personally order the tests, a message could appear informing the clinician, "This is a duplicate order." You could define the acceptable time limit for valid duplication, which would result in the message prompt. For example, chemistry profiles should be done one time per admission; electrolytes, one per day if on intravenous therapy. Nurses and/or unit clerks entering orders in the computer could see the message "duplication of test order" and override the order. However, many are reluctant to cancel or question the physician's orders. It is difficult to contact the ordering physician, who generally has left the unit before the orders are taken off the chart. In most organizations, physicians do not enter their orders or have the training required to view information of this nature on the monitor.

A study performed by the College of American Pathologists at 502 institutions showed 1.5% duplicate thyroid-stimulating hormone (TSH) orders within a period of 7 days. Ten percent of the institutions showed 4.5% or more of their orders duplicated. Nineteen percent of the physicians were unaware of the first order. In addition, 11% of the duplicate TSH assays performed in the laboratory had never been ordered by the physician. This conclusion supports our suggestion of computerized intervention. "Institutions aiming to reduce the frequency of duplicate testing should consider policies that decrease the opportunity for different physicians to order tests on a single patient and should increase the accuracy with which physician orders are transmitted to the laboratory" (33).

LESSON LEARNED

Communicating and eliminating duplicate orders would be most efficient if physicians personally entered their orders in the computer.

Phenytoin/Therapeutic Drug Monitoring

A group including pharmacists, clinicians, and laboratory workers established the indications for a serum phenytoin level.

INDICATIONS FOR SERUM LEVEL MONITORING

1. Check level after loading dose is given.
2. Check level for compliance of dosage.
3. Check if patient has signs of phenytoin toxicity.
4. Check if there is a new potential drug/drug or drug/nutrient interaction.
5. Check level after a change (dose or route).

After loading dose refers to sampling after reaching steady state. We also studied the timing of the phlebotomy draw (trough level 0–60 minutes before the next dose). If steady state has not been obtained, then the serum drug level is still rising. Decisions related to dosing could incorrectly assume a steady state, and an increase in dosage could result in elevated (toxic) levels. A steady state for phenytoin was defined as 5–7 days after an unchanged dose regimen (34). Other factors that can affect the level include drug/food and drug/drug interactions, variation in the severity of illness, stress, whether the person is lying down or standing up (increased patient plasma volume occurs in the prone position), age, weight, and diet (35).

Drug/Food, Drug/Drug Interactions

Tube feeding, vitamins (folate, vitamin D, and pyridoxine), antacids, H_2-antagonists, phenobarbital, carbamazepine, valproic acid, and antituberculosis drugs (e.g., isoniazid and rifampin).

Symptoms of Phenytoin Toxicity

Drowsiness, cortical dysfunction, visual blurring, incoordination, nystagmus, coma, and behavioral changes.

We found that 35% of phenytoin orders did not have a valid indication and 40% to 54% of the testing was done prior to reaching a steady state. Surprisingly, correct timing of the draw occurred only 30% of the time. There was minimum improvement despite three monitors over a 3-year period, communications through staff newsletters, and presentations at committees, including general staff meetings. Because of this we initiated clinical pharmacist involvement (Table 6-2). The pharmacist would be informed of all lab orders for serum phenytoin levels. If the patient had not reached study state, the pharmacist would call the doctor and would request involvement in regulating the dosage and monitoring drug levels. With successful intervention, we estimated a savings of $30,000/year related to lab charges. We felt the potential savings related to shortened stays and decreasing complications would be approximately $100,000 annually.

Review of the literature shows that our findings were not an isolated phenomenon. Therapeutic drug monitoring requires a knowledge of pharmacokinetics (how drug concentrations change in an individual patient with time) and pharmacodynamics (the effect of the drug in relationship to concentrations). Too often any unanticipated change in results is attributed to lab error. Steve Soldin performed a monitor of aminoglycosides that resulted in a decrease in the length of stay and number of toxic reactions in patients. This was due in part to an appropriate therapeutic drug monitoring imformation obtained before any testing was allowed. The forms required the amount of the drug to be given, the route of administration, and the time interval between when medication is given and when the blood is drawn. Some laboratories refuse to do the testing if needed information is unavailable. Others merely enter a comment that the timing of the draw may be inappropriate (36). Correcting issues related to therapeutic drug monitoring requires a more active approach than a comment on the chart.

Mason and Winters studied appropriate therapeutic drug monitoring and found that 68% of the sampling was not done during the study state (37). Bussey and Hoffman found that 43% of serum levels were inappropriately sampled. Furthermore, 40% of appropriately drawn serum levels were responded to inappropriately (38). Schoenenberger and others found only 27% had an appropriate indication (34). In addition, several studies identified clinical situations where monitoring was warranted but not performed (37,39). Wong and others found that 56% of phenytoin levels could not be justified on any grounds (40).

After initiating involvement of pharmacists with phenytoin ordering, a survey showed that only 6% of the tests were ordered inappropriately. This is a significant improvement. The testing order is not interfaced to pharmacy, and some are still drawn on the units before there can be pharmacist intervention. Also, some physicians do not want the pharmacist to write orders on their patients. Thus, there is room for additional improvement in the process.

In conclusion, improved accuracy of therapeutic drug monitoring is an area where we can improve patient care. The simple act of ordering a serum drug level does not guarantee that the information will be meaningful or useful. Both our experience with phenytoin and information in the literature support focusing efforts on improving monitoring of therapeutic drug levels, including not only phenytoin, but other frequently ordered therapeutic drug levels, such as digoxin, phenobarbital, and tegretol.

Warfarin

Complications related to anticoagulant therapy remain a significant clinical issue. This includes bleeding complications related to excessive dosing and thrombosis, such as deep vein or coronary thrombosis, related to less than optimal therapy (41). Adequate control of warfarin therapy diminishes the number of adverse events. This results in decreased costs related to fewer lab draws, office visits, and interventions associated with hospital and emergency department admission as well as rehabilitative services.

The therapeutic effect of warfarin is monitored by measuring the patient's prothrombin time (PT). The international normalized ratio (INR), which is used to monitor the patient's warfarin therapy, is an attempt to standardize prothrombin time results by multiplying the ratio of the patient's prothrombin time and the mean prothrombin time by a factor based on the sensitivity of the thromboplastin used. This is done because of the wide variation in the sensitivity of thromboplastin throughout the world and the United States. Wilt and colleagues predicted a potential cost savings of about $4,000 per year per patient for patients monitored by a pharmacist-managed anticoagulant service. These figures were based on $15 for the lab draw, $24 for testing, and a physician office visit cost of $37 to $86. Most of the cost savings were related to the additional costs of the emergency department and hospital admissions due to warfarin-related adverse events (42). Lee and Schommer demonstrated that patients managed by pharmacists had fewer hospital admissions than patients monitored by their physician. These results were a product of knowledge of the pharmacodynamics and pharmacokinetics of warfarin as well as close communication among the pharmacist, patient, and other significant health care providers (43).

Critical success factors for stabilization of a patient's warfarin therapy are close communication with the physician, quick access to PT/INR result, and the patient's level of understanding. These three issues play an important part in maintaining patients within an optimal therapeutic INR range appropriate to their disease state (44–49). A study addressing the patients' baseline knowledge of their therapy concluded that more time should be devoted to enhancing their knowledge of their therapy. Despite counseling during the hospital stay, after 3 months of additional counseling, improvement was noted (44). Patient knowledge apparently translates into compliance with dosing and earlier detection of complications (49). Macgregor and others, using pharmacists, had 84% of the INR results within a target range (±10%) at 6 months and 90% at 1 year. This is compared with 50% of the INRs previously within the desired range at the end of 1 year. There was increased patient satisfaction attributed in part to less waiting and more personal attention (50).

A sample of 87 patients admitted to Tucson Medical Center (TMC) during January and February of 1995 was identified as having a diagnosis of a disease state that required an-

TABLE 6-2. *Phenytoin monitoring process approved by TMC P & T Committee*

1. Order for phenytoin written.
2. Pharmacist receives order, evaluates and determines whether laboratory values[s] should be obtained.
   Indications for serum level monitoring include:
       Check level after loading dose is given.
       Check level for a newly admitted patient.
       Patient is symptomatic (i.e., Sz, symptoms of toxicity)
       Check if there is a drug/drug or drug/nutrient interaction.
3. Pharmacist writes note in chart re: dosing, loads, etc., and writes for appropriate lab[s].
   Sampling times for serum phenytoin levels:
       Loading dose
           Intravenous: 1.5–2 hours after end of infusion.
           Oral: 24 hours after loading dose.
       Maintenance dose
           Intravenous: 30 min before morning dose.
           Oral (divided): 30 min before morning dose.
           Oral (single): 30 min before scheduled dose.
4. If dosing, timing, etc. of phenytoin need to be changed in any way, then pharmacist contacts physician directly.
5. Once lab values are received and reviewed by the pharmacist, if there is need for physician intervention, the pharmacist will again contact the physician and write a note in the chart.
   Therapeutic level:
       10–20 µg/ml, but toxicity should be measured subjectively
       >100 µg/ml = lethal
       Interactions with test: ↑ by glucose, alkaline phosphatase ↓ by thyroxine, calcium

Adjust for low albumin and creatinine clearance greater than 25 ml/min:	Adjust for normal or low albumin and patient receiving dialysis:
Cp reported	Cp reported
CP normal binding =	CP normal binding =
[0.2] albumin − 0.1	[0.1] albumin − 0.1

   Dose adjustment:
   $$\frac{Dose \times CP\ desired}{Cp\ reported} = Dose\ desired$$
6. This ongoing process will take place throughout a patient's stay at TMC.

Phenytoin Dosing and Monitoring

Mechanism of action:
1. Stabilizes neuronal membranes by ↓ flow sodium ions across the cell membranes in the motor cortex.
2. Shortens the action potential of heart by prolonging the effective refractory period and suppressing the automaticity of ventricular pacemaker.

Indication:
1. Generalized tonic-clonic, simple partial and complex partial seizures.
2. Prevention of Sz following head trauma/neurosurgery.
3. Ventricular arrhythmias, including those associated with digitalis intoxication, prolonged Q-T interval, and surgical repair of congenital heart diseases in children.
4. Epidermolysis bullosa.

Contraindications:
1. Hypersensitivity to phenytoin and other hydantoins
2. Heart block, sinus bradycardia

Warnings/precautions:
1. May ↑ frequency of absence Sz.
2. IV form may cause hypotension and skin necrosis at IV site of small veins.
3. Pts having porphyria

TABLE 6-2. *(Continued)*

4. Caution in patients having hepatic dysfunction, sinus bradycardia, S-A block, A-V block, or hepatic impairment.

Symptoms of toxicity:
Unsteady gait, slurred speech, confusion, nausea, hypothermia, fever, hypotension, respiratory depression, and coma.

Drug interactions:
↑ effect with:
Rifampicin, cisplatin, vinblastine, bleomycin, folic acid; binds with enteral feedings. Tube feedings should be held 1° before and after each dose, and tubing should be flushed with 20 ml of sterile water before and after dose.
↑ effect with:
Cimetidine, chloramphenicol, isoniazid, trimethoprim, sulfonamides
↑ toxicity of:
Valproic acid, ethosuximide, primidone, warfarin, oral contraceptives, corticosteroids, cyclosporine, theophylline chloramphenicol, rifampicin, doxycycline, quinidine, mexiletine, disopyramide, dopamine, nondepolarizing skeletal muscle

Kinetic Parameters of Phenytoin
Volume of distribution; Vd
Neonates:
Premature: 1–1.2 L/kg
Full term: 0.8–0.9 L/kg
and

Infants: 0.7–0.8 L/kg
Children: 0.7 L/kg
Adults: 0.6–0.7 L/kg
Time to reach peak serum concentration (Cp):
Oral formulations:
Extended-release capsule: 4–12 hr
Immediate-release preparation: 2–3 hr

Dosing
Intravenous:
All: Loading dose (LD); 15–20 mg/kg
mg/kg
Rate: <18 yrs: 1–8 mg/kg^{-1} min^{-1}
Maintenance dose: start 24 hr after LD
Neonates (<4 wks); 3–5 mg/kg^{-1} day^{-1}
4 wks and up; 4–8 mg/kg^{-1} day^{-1}
or
>18 yrs: 50 mg/min
Protein binding:
Adults: 90–95%
↓ in patients with ↑ bilirubin, urea, and ↑ albumin; up to 20% in neonates
15% in infants toxicity
Metabolism:
Metabolized in the liver having dose-dependent pharmacokinetics
Elimination:
Eliminated by the kidneys

Loading and Maintenance
Oral:
LD: same as IV but given in 5 increments every 2 hr until total dose administered
Maintenance: start 24 hr after LD
Divide total daily dose over 12-, 8-, 6-hr intervals. Adults may be given extended-release 300 mg qHS.

ticoagulation therapy. This sample identified 10 patients who experienced an adverse event related to oral anticoagulant therapy over the course of treatment at TMC. A conservative cost of treatment for these adverse events totaled approximately $64,000. Projected potential savings for the payer would be approximately $384,000/year. This does not include additional costs accumulated outside the TMC facility, the emotional effect, or the costs of time off from work accumulated by the family or patient. We presently are using a clinical pharmacology intervention with a defined pathway focused on several different clinical offices and hospital nursing units (Fig. 6-4).

The Couma-Care software with a pharmacist intervention was used on a trial basis at a busy internal medicine office. The results were excellent. Data are now being compiled in a cooperative five-hospital study for later publication. However, the physicians from

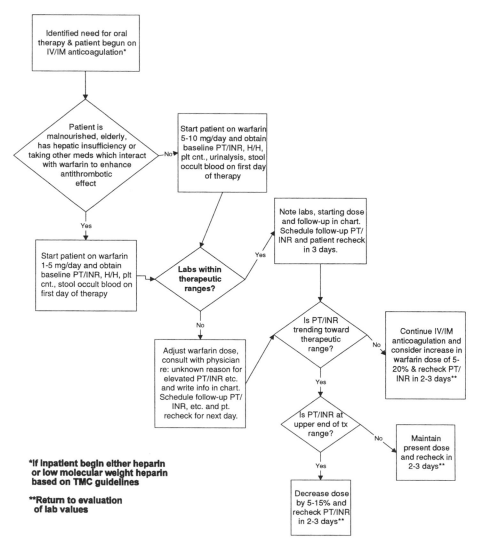

FIG 6-4. Algorithm for regulation of oral anticoagulant utilization by clinical pharmacologists.

the office who had tried Couma-Care were unwilling to submit their patients as controls because their prior experience was so positive.

KEY ELEMENTS

Patient characteristics
Patient compliance
Diet
Drug/drug interaction
Drug/food interaction
Other illnesses or comorbidity
Timely lab results with therapeutic response
Patient education
Accurate measurement of adverse events

This warfarin dosing/monitor that we used is based on a number of well-researched articles (51–60) (Table 6-3). The leadership for this protocol was provided by Teresa Nord and Mike Melby. There are two dosing protocols. The first is for low-intensity warfarin therapy used for deep vein thrombosis, venous thromboembolism in patients with atrial fibrillation, valvular heart disease, bioprosthetic heart valves, or acute myocardial infarction. Many would argue that deep vein thrombosis can now be treated on an outpa-

TABLE 6-3. *Warfarin dosing/monitoring protocol*

Therapeutic Goal of INR of 2.0–3.0	Dose	Therapeutic Goal of INR 2.5–3.5	Dose
Day 1		Day 1	
Patient work-up unremarkable	10 mg	Patient work-up unremarkable	10 mg
Patient at risk of hemorrhage	7.5 mg	Patient at risk of hemorrhage (recommend use of lower range)	7.5mg
Day 2		Day 2	
No change in patient	10 mg	No change in patient	10 mg
Patient subtherapeutic	7.5 mg	Patient subtherapeutic	7.5 mg
Patient therapeutic	5.0 mg	Patient therapeutic (go to day 5+)	5.0 mg
Patient supratherapeutic	Hold	Patient supratherapeutic (INR <3.7) (go to day 5+)	2.5 mg
			Hold
		Patient supratherapeutic (INR >3.7)	
Day 3		Day 3	
No change in patient	10 mg	No change in patient	10 mg
Patient subtherapeutic	7.5 mg	Patient subtherapeutic	7.5 mg
Patient therapeutic	5.0 mg	Patient therapeutic	7.5 mg
Patient supratherapeutic	Hold	Patient supratherapeutic (INR <3.7)	2.5 mg
Dose held previous day	2.5 mg	Patient supratherapeutic (INR >3.7)	2.5 mg
		Dose held previous day	
Day 4		Day 4	
Patient subtherapeutic	5.0 mg	Patient subtherapeutic	7.5 mg
Patient therapeutic	5.0 mg	Patient therapeutic	7.5 mg
Patient supratherapeutic (INR <3.3)	2.5 mg	Patient supratherapeutic (INR <3.7)	5.0 mg
Patient supratherapeutic (INR >3.3)	Hold	Patient supratherapeutic (INR >3.7)	Hold
Dose held previous day	2.5 mg	Dose held previous day	5.0 mg
Day 5+		Day 5+	
Patient subtherapeutic	↑ by 2.5 mg	Patient subtherapeutic	↑ by 2.5 mg
Patient therapeutic	Same dose	Patient therapeutic	Same dose
Patient supratherapeutic (INR <3.3)	↓ by 1.25 mg	Patient supratherapeutic (INR <3.7)	↓ by 2.0 mg
Patient supratherapeutic (INR <3.5)	↓ by 2.25 mg	Patient supratherapeutic (INR >3.7)	Hold
Patient supratherapeutic (INR >3.5)	Hold	Dose held previous day	5.0 mg
Dose held previous day	2.5 mg		

tient basis with low-molecular-weight heparin, but at present this is in the trial stages at many institutions, including ours. This dosing protocol's goal is an INR between 2.0 and 3.0. The second protocol is used for patients with mechanical prosthetic valves and for those with recurrent systemic embolism. In this protocol the goal is an INR of 2.5–3.5.

Smaller starting doses should be used for patients who are malnourished, are elderly, have a smaller than average blood volume for distribution, or are taking medications that cannot be discontinued and that interact with warfarin to enhance the antithrombotic effect. Part of the pharmacist's role is to continue to monitor carefully for adverse events as well as to adjust the warfarin dosing.

Urine Cultures

Urinalysis by the dipstick method or urinalysis with microscopic analysis can be used as a screen for urine cultures. Findings of white blood cells or bacteria are valid indications for urine culture. Although there are some indications for urine cultures in the absence of abnormal findings on urinalysis, they are definitely the exception to the rule and should be infrequent. One example would be a patient who is symptomatic for urinary tract infection and is immunocompromised (e.g., an AIDS patient or patients undergoing chemotherapy). If your standard order is urinalysis, culture if indicated, it will eliminate a number of needless cultures and unnecessary costs.

The following is a study performed at TMC by the Infection Control Department by Sandy Baus, Infection Control Manager, Barry Friedman, Infectious Disease Consultant.

Results

All urine specimens were cultured for the data analysis followed by chart review to determine the rationale for the order.

CONCLUSIONS

1. When collected properly, a urinalysis and culture, if indicated, is an appropriate test. All patients who might have had a urinary tract infection were identified using this protocol.
2. Urine cultures done while patients are on broad-spectrum antibiotics are likely to be negative. Concentration of antibiotics in the urine is usually so high that even growth of resistant organisms may be inhibited.
3. When patients are not on antibiotics, a urine specimen with a negative urinalysis is unlikely to grow organisms.
4. A false-positive result occurred in one specimen. That specimen grew mixed flora, suggesting contamination as a result of poor collection technique.
5. A mini-cath urine specimen collected from females is likely to provide more accurate results than the so-called clean-cath mid-stream urine specimen.

Recommendation: Order urinalysis culture if indicated for all patients, unless specific underlying conditions suggest otherwise (e.g., a severely immunocompromised individual).

In a study that included a review of charts looking for literature-based exclusion criteria for urine cultures, approximately 15% of the cultures were not indicated. Chart reviews are always tedious, but additional education or development of a clinical pathway for urinary cultures could prove rewarding (61).

TABLE 6-4. *Urinalysis orders/culture results*

Type ordered by physician	Total number (44)	Sub number	Results
Urine culture only	4/44	4/4	No growth
		3/4	Had received antibiotics within 24 hr
		3/4	On antibiotics at the time specimen collected
Urinalysis and culture	10/44	6/10	Culture not indicated
		5/6	No growth
		1/6	Mixed flora (probable contaminant)
		4/10	Culture indicated based on urinalysis
		2/4	Single organism with greater than 10^5 microorganisms
		1/4	Cath specimen—IV antibiotic given 24 hr prior to culture
		1/4	Multiple organisms—Quadriplegic patient
Urinalysis—culture if indicated	30/44	30/30	Had normal urinalysis and no growth

A follow-up study performed after approximately 6 months showed 51% of the urines ordered with a request for culture. Of those with a urinalysis, only 11 or (18%) had findings that would have reflexed to a culture (if ordered as urinalysis culture). Of those ordered as a culture and urinalysis with a negative urinalysis, one had a positive culture (*Enterococcus*). Information on the method of collection was not provided. This specimen was from a female with stress incontinence. *Enterococcus* is a potential contaminant because of its ubiquitous nature (62).

In conclusion, we have to pursue this with a different approach. Providing information without active intervention has not succeeded. Potential steps that are under consideration include the following:

1. Eliminate all orders other than urinalysis; culture if indicated. This would presumably not be acceptable to the clinicians without significant campaigning. This would include not only going to committees but publishing data regularly to support the change. The preceding data would support that recommendation. We did this at a small peripheral hospital where 22 out of 25 cultures for urine were positive. The three negative cultures were ordered by physicians who were consultants. Clinicians felt there was no negative clinical impact to this change in their ordering process.
2. Perform a urinalysis on each culture ordered only as urine culture. This could provide useful feedback to the clinicians.
3. Add an appropriate message where indicated. For example, "This negative urine culture was associated with a negative urinalysis."
4. Contact each physician who orders a urine culture without urinalysis. The numbers make this an unrealistic goal if we want one of the pathologists to dialogue with the physician. We could either send a letter that includes data or send a letter and call selective doctors who have the highest number of variations. This seems realistic and is most likely to gain acceptance.

ISTAT Usage

We have utilized ISTAT bedside testing on our trauma services for several years. (ISTAT is a hand-held instrument for bedside testing that can measure sodium, potassium, chloride, hemoglobin, hematocrit, glucose, calcium, and magnesium. Specific test selection is determined by the cartridge used.) If the ISTAT done at the bedside included a sodium, potassium, chloride, hematocrit, hemoglobin, and glucose, then it would be duplication to order a chemistry profile and a complete blood count (assuming your primary concern was the hemoglobin and hematocrit) at the same time. We noted a significant (25%) duplication of testing. On questioning the doctors, we found that it was related not to their orders, but to the fact that in triaging trauma patients a certain amount of blood was drawn on admission to the emergency department. If the doctors had left without writing specific orders for the lab, it was assumed that they wanted the standard testing sent to the laboratory. The duplications were based on nurse assumptions related to a historically outdated process. Our initial assessment that this was a doctor-related duplication was incorrect. The process has been changed and corrected.

LESSONS LEARNED

Observe the entire process before drawing conclusions.
Data impacts belief systems and can change behavior.

Pap Smears

The American College of Obstetrics and Gynecology has suggested certain guidelines for Pap smears: "The US Preventative Task Force recommended in 1989 that the time interval between smears should be 1–3 years, depending on the presence of risk factors for cervical cancer. The risk of an abnormality occurring within 3–5 years after three consecutive negative annual smears is minimum in low-risk patients" (63). "The cost-effectiveness of cytologic screening for vaginal neoplasm after removal of the cervix for benign disease has not been demonstrated." In consideration of the low risk of preinvasive vaginal lesions or invasive cancer, however, periodic cytologic evaluation of the vagina, based on the patient's risk factors, is suggested (64).

If the patient is at low risk and has had three normal Pap smears, then there is no need for an annual Pap smear. A Pap smear every 2–3 years is sufficient.

Pal Evans, an obstetrician and gynecologist, as well as medical director of TMC health care, became interested in the subject and developed into its champion. His initial goal was appropriate use of cytology screening in women more than 50 years of age with no cervix and no history of dysplasia, endometrial, or cervical cancer. In these patients, testing can be performed every 3 years or at the physician's discretion. This is a sensitive area, because the system is interested in structure, related to more cost efficiency, and physicians are interested in autonomy in handling their patients. Education and data are necessary for doctors and patients if we are to change the process. Their goal is demonstrated in the mission statement.

MISSION STATEMENT

Our mission is to educate physicians, other providers, and patients about the appropriate use of cytology screening in women more than 50 years of age who have no cervix and no history of dysplasia or endometrial or cervical cancer.

Random sampling of Pap smear results in women more than 50 years of age showed that approximately 23% had a hysterectomy, 4% had a history of an abnormal Pap smear, and 2% had current, new abnormal findings on Pap smears. Thus 71% of the patients would have no need of an additional Pap smear for 3 years, and the 23% who had a hysterectomy would not need another Pap smear if no vaginal cuff abnormalities were noted clinically. The algorithm (see Fig. 6-5) was distributed and an intensive education program was initiated for OB/GYN physicians, nurse midwives, and primary care physicians. Shortly thereafter there was an initial 10% decrease in Pap smears in women over 50 (see Fig. 6-6). Individual physicians will be given follow-up data on a periodic basis. The following announcement was also sent out:

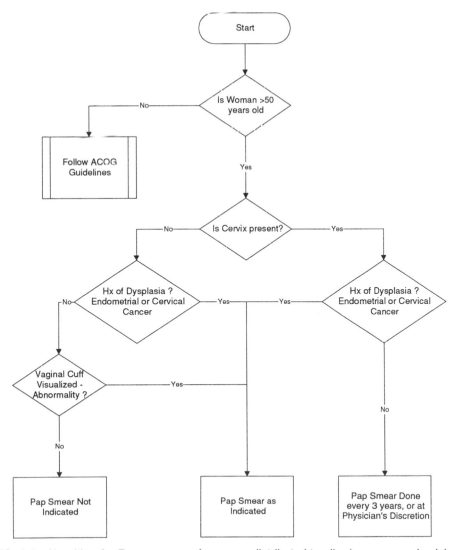

FIG. 6-5. Algorithm for Pap smear performance distributed to all primary care physicians.

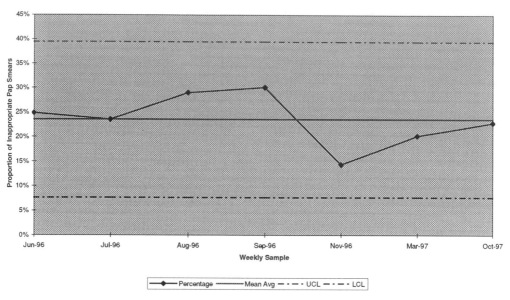

FIG. 6-6. Control chart showing a decrease in the number of inappropriate Pap smears.

Pap Smears

One less thing to worry about...

If you have had a hysterectomy and have never had an abnormal Pap smear, cervical or endometrial cancer, Pap smears are unnecessary.

Pap smears are used to detect cancer of the cervix. Because vaginal cancer is extremely rare and hysterectomies remove the uterus and cervix, Pap smears have been found to be unnecessary in this population. This data was reported in *The New England Journal of Medicine*, Nov. 21, 1996.

Regular gynecological examinations are still necessary for all women, regardless of whether they need Pap smears. For more information, talk to your gynecologist or your primary care physician.

There was also a significant drop in the number of Pap smears for all ages.

Standing Orders

Standing orders assume that patients are basically the same, and when used in a reflex manner can result in excess testing. In reviewing simple, uncomplicated births (vaginal deliveries) at our hospital there were more than thirty different sets of standard orders with a significant amount of variation. For example, Dr. Brown would not write specific orders, but merely used standing orders, which he had previously selected for all uncomplicated deliveries or used the same standing orders and added several orders for a more complicated delivery.

The Department of Obstetrics and Gynecology had a champion, Sherry Maloney, for the process of reducing standard orders. She took this on as a project with help from several key physicians and tenaciously worked to develop and win acceptance of the pathways. Eight months of ordering data were collected from uncomplicated deliveries, post c-section orders, post vaginal deliveries, and post simple hysterectomies. The most common orders were tabulated and presented to a select group. After their approval, the "common" standard orders were posted and mailed to a select few, who used the hospital infrequently, and comments were requested. The final potential consensus orders went to the obstetric/gynecologic committee for approval. These orders could be altered as needed by crossing out or adding orders.

All but a few accepted the pathways; those who did not continued to write their own orders. Now no standing orders were available. One of the positive changes included simplification of pharmacy orders. With less variation there was greater familiarity with the orders and less opportunity to carry them out incorrectly. The only remaining postoperative lab order, done on the first post-op date, was a complete blood count. Previously, many of the clinicians had ordered this test each post-op day. Simple things that took time, such as abdominal binders, were eliminated, saving time for the staff without compromising care. The cost savings in lab and pharmacy have not been great, but the nurses have received the elimination of variation in patient care and feel that, because of the standardization of their patient care routines, they are giving better care.

Standing orders are of value to physicians and patients if they are reached by consensus and represent the latest scientific thinking combined with what has been learned through the experience of the local clinicians. Obviously, there are exceptions to following these standing orders, but they should be in the minority. Hospitals that support the use of standing orders are in a position to promote patient-specific orders that would be more cost-effective.

A hospital in Orlando, Florida, eliminated standing orders and curtailed lab and other diagnostic testing by 2%. The biggest hurdle was "having the guts to do it" (65). In one study standing orders were prohibited for a time. During that time, test volumes decreased by 55%, and test outliers decreased by 95%. Analysis of the data showed many orders that were routinely repeated, unrelated to previous test values. Periodic publication of the data on individual physician usage as a means of peer comparison had a role in this process change (66).

We have successfully initiated changes in the obstetric/gynecologic areas that we hope to initiate in other areas. The major requirement is a tenacious, data-driven champion.

Stools for Ova and Parasites/Stool Leukocytes

There is no need to do stools for ova and parasites if the patient has been hospitalized for more than 3 days before symptomatology. If the study is indicated, one specimen is adequate (67). If more than one specimen is submitted, we are presently combining specimens, giving a single result, and dialoguing with the ordering physician. This was done by Dr. Sparks, who uses the opportunity for continuing education of clinicians on the laboratory's recommendations related to diarrhea.

At the University of Iowa more than 2,000 examinations were done each year for ova and parasites; they had a yield of less than 0.5%, of which half were nonpathogenic parasites. By the criteria mentioned earlier, they eliminated two-thirds of the requests. They also extended the same criteria to stool cultures for bacteria and questioned the value of testing for stool leukocytes. The absence or presence of leukocytes in the stool did not correlate well with gastrointestinal pathology. We eliminated the test for stool leukocytes more than a year ago with no negative repercussions (68). However, this elimination did result in a number of discussions with clinicians.

Microbiology Culture Results and Communication with Pharmacy

Improved communication with pharmacy about microbiology culture correlated with antibiotic sensitivities represents an opportunity not only to ensure efficacy of the prescribed antibiotic but to compare relative costs of potential treatments. We have found antibiotics being prescribed that are both more expensive than necessary and resistant to the organism. An additional concern was the amount of incorrect dosing of antibiotics. Optimum dosing has an obvious potential to affect patient care positively. One of the obstacles to this process is lack of good communication between the pharmacy and lab. However, interfaces exist that greatly facilitate the process. Some institutions also use the same software for both the pharmacy and the lab, which allows easy exchange of information between the two sites.

We have initiated a software change in the report format that communicates resistance or sensitivity of each positive culture for various antibiotics and comparative costs of treatment, as well as proper dosage information (see Table 6-5). This will be used for both outpatients and inpatients. The advantage of this is consistent, ongoing information readily available to the clinician.

Clinical Practice Guidelines/Hepatitis C

Financial pressures in health care, rapid development of new technology, and data supporting inappropriate care have given strong support to the strategy of developing prac-

---

TABLE 6-5. *Tucson Medical Center Chart with Susceptibility/Dosage/Cost Data*

Unit:	0300	Room: 0308-1
	11/13/97	Page: 1
Name:	DOE, JANE A.	86Y F
	M-R #: 000001122334	
Admitting Dr:	SMITH, JOHN A., MD	
	Acct #: 1122334	
	Admit:	
	01/01/1997	

URINE CULT/CLEAN CATCH OR CATH   STATUS: FNL 01/02/97
COLLECTION DATE/TIME: 01/01/97   1100
ACCESSION NO: M11111
  SPECIMEN DESCRIPTION: CATHETERIZED URINE
  ADDITIONAL INFORMATION: NONE
  CULTURE   1. >100,000 CFU/ML KLEBSIELLA PNEUMONIAE

SUSCEPTIBILITY

1. >100,000 CFU/ML KLEBSIELLA PNEUMONIAE

Drug	MIC—UG/ML	Interpretation			
	Route — Dosage — IP Cost		Op Cost / Day		
AMPICILLIN	>=32	RESISTANT	V 2.0 g, ×4	$ 7.09	na
			PO 250 mg, ×4	$ 0.22	$ 0.68
1ST GEN. CEPHALOSPOR	<=2	SUSCEPTIBLE	IM, 1.0 G, ×3	$ 3.44	na
			IV 1.0 g, ×3	$ 3.44	na
GENTAMICIN	<=.5	SUSCEPTIBLE	IM 210–350 mg	$ 0.90	na
			IV 210–350	$ 0.90	na
NITROFURANTOIN	<=32	SUSCEPTIBLE	PO 100 mg, ×4	$ 2.17	$ 4.69
TRIMETH-SULFAMETHOXA	<=10	SUSCEPTIBLE	IV 160TMP/800 SMX	$ 1.69	na
			PO 1 DS Tab, ×2	$ 0.11	$ 1.25

CLINICAL LABORATORY DIR. PAUL D. BOZZO M.D.
  M-R #: 0000011122334
P. O. BOX 42195 TUCSON, AZ 85733
  Acct #: 1122334
Phone: 520-325-5310
  NAME: DOE, JANE A.
  0308-01   PAGE: 1   LOC:

tice guidelines (also referred to as practice parameters or clinical pathways [69,70]). The goal is to offer health care providers the most efficient and cost-effective processes, which will improve outcomes, including patient and physician satisfaction. Insurance companies and independent research organizations such as RAND have a goal of reducing geographic variation in practice patterns and more effective use of health care resources (71). These pathways are formally developed to assist the practitioner in determination of care in specific clinical conditions. Congress, physicians, health providers, and payers have all focused on practice parameters as a means of achieving that goal. Congress provided funds for the Agency for Health Care Policy and Research to coordinate a national research program and establish a databank to support development of practice parameters (72). Those developing parameters should take into account appropriateness, asking themselves whether each step contributes to the patient's outcome. If it does, they should determine whether the health benefit of each step exceeds the health risk by a sufficient margin to make it worthwhile. Pathways are a combination of the recommendations from the medical literature, clinical expertise that is supportable, and a consensus of the local design group. Theoretically, pathways should improve quality and eventually lower costs because of improved outcomes. Some data relating the effect of using pathways on outcomes are presently available to support their use, but this information is not as prominent in the literature as pathways published without good measurements to prove their worth (73,74). Hopefully, more outcome-related studies will be forthcoming in the near future. Even though the data support is minimal, the concept is worthwhile. Using clinical pathways in your organization for processes with a good deal of variation can produce consensus action guidelines that can improve the quality of care. Laboratory testing is common to most pathways. Thus laboratory workers are in a position to be leaders in this area.

In selecting which pathway to develop consider the following:

High volume
High cost
Problem-prone areas
Critical issues
Easily solvable problems

As with other quality issues, participation from all disciplines involved is crucial. The measurement of outcomes can be used to judge success of efforts. Outcomes can be measured in four areas: clinical, functional, satisfaction, and costs. Clinical measures include infection rates, appropriate admissions, mortality, and morbidity; functional measures include readmissions, physical function, mental health, ability to work or return to school, and pain. Determining satisfaction requires a valid measurement by trained surveyors or patients, physicians, and staff. Cost is one aspect of outcome presently available to most health care institutions (75). Outcomes are best examined not only in the present, but also in the future (e.g., 6 months to 1 year after the encounter). A key success factor in physician acceptance is whether the recommendations are viewed as an aid in helping to provide improved care to their patients. If the doctors do not follow the protocols, their development is a waste of time and money. Physician participation in selecting and developing the protocols is critical to gaining acceptance. Development of a protocol obligates follow-up with data feedback to participants. Blue Cross/Blue Shield of Oregon has successfully encouraged participation by providing financial rewards for those who follow the guidelines (76). Acceptance comes from the belief that the pathway is worthwhile. For this to occur, the process must not be seen as another hassle factor for management.

We did a clinical pathway for hepatitis C testing in which the starting point was a positive test for antibody to hepatitis C using the enzyme-linked immunosorbent assay (ELISA) technique. The ELISA technique is not as specific as the more expensive polymerase chain reaction testing for ribonucleic acid (RNA). The lab testing is expensive, but even more costly is interferon treatment, which can be more than $10,000 and result in a sustained response in less than 20% of the treated patients (77).

Before interferon treatment is considered, the patient must have a positive qualitative polymerase chain reaction (PCR) RNA and/or a liver biopsy. Although both tests indicate ongoing viral duplication, a PCR-RNA qualitative is significantly less expensive than a PCR-RNA quantitative. The approaches to a symptomatic patient, an asymptomatic blood donor, a patient with acute hepatitis and a patient with chronic hepatitis are different (Figs. 6-7, 6-8, 6-9). The consensus was to follow patients if they have a normal liver function test and to follow this test with a hepatitis C PCR-RNA qualitative if the enzymes become abnormal. This procedure is being debated because it is known that some patients have active hepatitis C and normal liver function tests. The consensus was that hepatitis C PCR-RNA qualitative is the ultimate test.

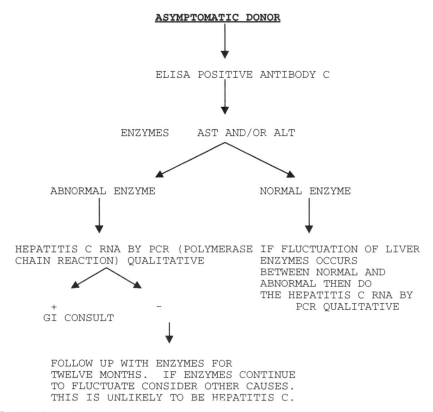

FIG. 6-7. Algorithm for follow-up of ELISA-positive antibody C in asymptomatic donors.

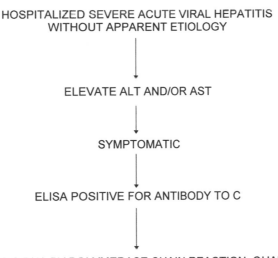

FIG. 6-8. Algorithm for follow-up of ELISA-positive antibody C in hospitalized severely ill acute hepatitis patients without apparent etiology.

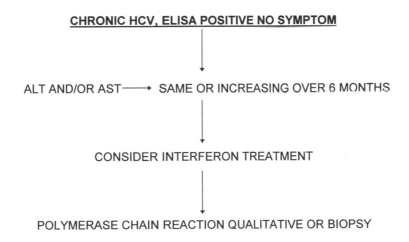

NOTE: PCR POSITIVE REQUIRED FOR TREATMENT. LIVER BIOPSY MAY BE REQUIRED TO DETERMINE TRUE STATUS

FIG. 6-9. Algorithm for ELISA-positive antibody follow-up in patients who are asymptomatic but have a long-term history of abnormal ELISA tests for hepatitis C or abnormal liver function studies.

The following is a newsletter which I wrote with input from other committee members that discusses clinical pathways for hepatitis C:

Position Paper: Hepatitis C (March, 1997)

Hepatitis C causes a type of viral hepatitis that is not distinguishable by clinical presentation or liver function tests from other causes of acute hepatitis. Liver biopsy histologic pattern is not specific but hepatitis C is more *likely* to have heavy lymphoid aggregates, fatty change of liver, and bile duct injury.

Diagnosis depends on demonstrating a positive serological assay. The ELISA testing unassociated with elevated liver enzymes should be confirmed by an assay for HCV RNA. In most instances, RIBA positivity (indicating the presence of virus) correlates well with a positive HCV RNA polymerase chain reaction that correlates with viral replication.

HCV RNA is readily detected in the serum of infected individuals at lower concentration than hepatitis B. Hepatitis HCV concentrations in other body fluids (e.g., saliva, semen, urine, stool, and vaginal secretions) are even lower or undetectable. HCV is less likely than HVB to be spread via perinatal or sexual contact or among family members. HCV is a frequent complication of intravenous drug abuse, renal dialysis patients, recipients of untreated commercial preparations of clotting factor concentrations, and those receiving an organ transplant. HCV is the major cause of posttransfusion hepatitis.

Hepatitis C has an incubation period of 5–7 weeks; aminotransferase activities rise and clinical manifestations become evident at this time. First-generation immunoassays, such as ELISA, become positive at approximately 12 weeks. Second-generation assays, such as RIBA or HCV RNA, may become positive as early as 2 weeks but more often at 5–6 weeks. Hepatitis C has a much greater propensity to become chronic (lasting greater than 6 months) than hepatitis B. Persisting HCV infections may be present in a patient despite normalization of liver enzyme activity.

Course of Disease. Hepatitis C exhibits an intermittent course with episodes of increased symptoms and laboratory abnormalities separated by periods of relative quiescence. In long-term studies, 25% to 50% progressed to cirrhosis, and approximately 50% of this population will develop hepatocellular carcinoma, depending on the timing. However, the literature reflects a screened population. Hepatocellular carcinoma may take more than 30 years to develop.

Approximately 45% respond to interferon therapy but still may experience recurrences. Approximately 33% are totally responsive to treatment with interferon. Treatment is complex and expensive requiring subcutaneous injections over a prolonged period of time. The latest outcome studies used higher doses and longer treatment.

Our goal is to adopt a consensus clinical pathway for appropriate hepatitis C testing. In reviewing test orders, there is considerable variation in the approach. After reviewing the literature, the attached protocol related to hepatitis C was developed by a group including general internists, one pathologist, and several gastroenterologists.

Direct any questions to Paul Bozzo, M.D., 520-324-1938.

Suggested Exam (sent with the newsletter)

1. *Question:* What is the first test(s) that should be ordered when there are consistent abnormalities of liver function and hepatitis is suspect?
   Answer: Hepatitis screens that include hepatitis B surface antigen, B surface antibody, hepatitis core antibody, hepatitis A (high immunoglobulin G [IgG] followed by immunoglobulin M [IgM] when the IgG is positive), and hepatitis C antibody by ELISA.

2. *Question:* What are the key questions you want to answer for the patient?
   Answer: Do you have hepatitis infection now? Do you need treatment?

3. *Question:* What single test is best for answering this question?
   Answer: Both of the answers to question 2 require a positive hepatitis C by RNA-PCR qualitative. The determination of treatment requires additional clinical information and possibly liver biopsy.

4. *Question:* When is the RIBA test indicated?

Answer: It is not, because it does not indicate viral duplication, which implies activity. RIBA tests for anti-HCV, so it detects the body's response to HCV. RIBA negative tells you that the ELISA test for C may be a false positive, which occurs approximately 3% to 5% of the time.

5. *Question:* Does a positive HCV RNA PCR qualitative indicate activity?
   Answer: Yes, it means you have circulating HCV and replication of virus, but it does not distinguish between progressive and nonprogressive liver disease.

6. *Question:* Does HCV RNA PCR qualitative positive mean the patient will be treated?
   Answer: No, it merely means that the patient has viremia.

7. *Question:* What constitutes cause for treatment?
   Answer: Although there are several schools of thought, all would agree that evidence of progressive liver disease is required, probably best determined by evidence of active necrosis in liver biopsies.

Suggested Steps in Developing a Pathway

1. Select a topic. Prioritize to make sure you get the most bang for your buck.
2. Form a committee to work on pathway. The physician or nurse leader should call personally to discuss the proposed project and obtain commitment. Include respected champions in the specialty who are most intimate with the pathway. Include specialists, primary care physicians, and other health care providers involved in the process.
3. Review the literature. Send key articles to committee members.
4. Write an initial rough draft to use as a nidus for discussion.
5. Convene the committee. Send results of the meeting and discuss with all committee members, whether present or not; ask for feedback.
6. Reconvene to review and hopefully reach a consensus decision.
7. Disseminate the final pathway to staff and post on the nursing units. Consider including (a) a position statement; (b) a short, related quiz; (c) a request for feedback.
8. Measure the impact of the pathway on patient outcome.

Physicians' buy-in remains the first priority if pathways are to be successful. One approach, which others have used successfully, is to convene a second group that is an expansion of the first group to have a larger nidus that will accept the concept. If you meet a good deal of opposition, this could be a signal for the initial group to reconvene and reconsider areas of concern or focus education on particular points.

Convening the initial group, which included some of the key gastroenterologists in the community, to develop the hepatitis C pathway resulted in a 66% decrease in what was considered inappropriate hepatitis C testing before we published the pathway. Consults and discussions involving the primary group disseminated the information and resulted in decreased testing before the pathway was officially published. Since then we have published the pathways and, with continuing discussions, have had requests to redistribute the information again. A year later I am still receiving positive feedback on the utilization of this pathway.

One of the ongoing issues is development of a feasible system where guidelines can be triggered and used. A diagnosis, chief complaint, or esoteric lab test request could trigger the appearance of the algorithm on a monitor for the clinician's review. This would also facilitate tracking of outcome data for those patients where the protocol was followed. Some organizations make the pathway part of the chart. The clinical diagnosis triggers the placing of the protocol on the chart. Others merely keep the protocols in a notebook on the nursing units (76). User-friendly, timely information, provided simultaneously with the clinician writing orders, is essential.

Additional Pathways

Pathways can result in cost savings and improved care. We've done this in a large number of areas, including asthma, prostate cancer, diabetes mellitus, back pain, and screening for breast cancer. In a select group of people with diabetes mellitus, an ongoing graphic representation of their fasting blood sugar levels tabulated by the patient resulted in greater compliance (smaller standard deviation of fasting blood sugars). We feel that improved compliance was related to having the graph as a visual aid. It is easier to comply with the process when you can see progressive improvement. This study was initiated after a presentation by Brent James of a similar successful process at InterMountain Health. Our process illustrates the need for a champion with some passion to make a pathway work. The initial champion moved out of town, and the use of guidelines disappeared until another champion assumed responsibility and accountability.

Test Utilization

Laboratory workers are under pressure to reduce the number of lab tests. A major concern is the potential for test reduction to affect the quality of care negatively. Even when the number of lab tests is reduced by as much as 67%, investigators have not seen a negative effect on clinical decisions (78). In one study, practice guidelines were designated for a series of specific medical problems. In the subsequent 12 months lab tests decreased by almost 21%, but outcomes judged by readmission rates and mortality were unaffected (79). If we are to modify behavior and thereby reduce testing, we must present relevant information to the clinician. Various approaches have been tried, including defining the suggested frequency of testing. For example, if potassium tests as normal and the patient is not on intravenous feedings, than only one potassium test should be ordered per day (80). This behavior is easier to modify in an academic situation involving residents, who have not developed criteria for testing ingrained by years of personal experience (81–83).

We periodically send data on utilization of outpatient laboratory tests related to managed care to groups of physicians (family practice, pediatrics, internal medicine, and obstetrics). A line graph (Fig. 6-10) shows their test frequency compared with peers based on number of tests and costs (Fig. 6-11) A histogram shows their test selection pattern compared with peers (Fig. 6-12). The individual provider is the only one to know his number on the line graph.

It is important to provide information on test utilization without indicating right or wrong. However, the implication is that increased usage is less desirable. The individual awareness of practice patterns compared with peers has changed test utilization for some physicians. They look at peers who have a successful practice and order fewer diagnostic tests. It raises the question, "Am I getting any significant information from additional testing?" At the request of the involved physicians, we are beginning to provide additional information, including gender distribution and average age. This information addresses the initial response of most physicians when reviewing the data, namely: "My practice makeup is different." We found no significant differences in average age or gender among the specialties surveyed.

We have started to meet with groups of physicians to discuss test utilization. They have expressed an interest in more information about selective tests. The focus was on those tests

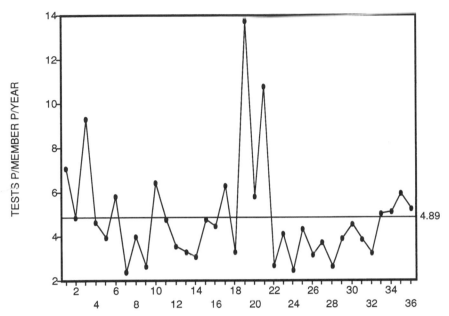

FIG. 6-10. Each dot on the chart represents the utilization of laboratory tests per assigned life per year in an internist's practice. Only the individual physician is aware of his or her number on comparison data; 4.89 is the average utilization for this group of physicians. Test utilization per member per year = 6.32.

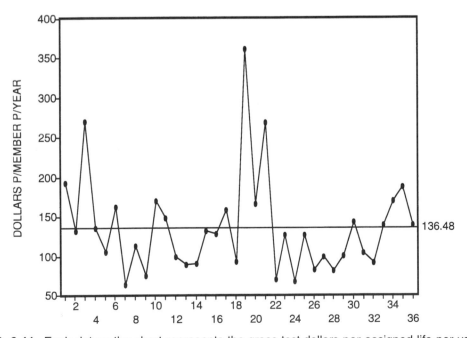

FIG. 6-11. Each dot on the chart represents the gross test dollars per assigned life per year in an internist's practice. Only the individual physician is aware of his or her number on the comparison data; $136.48 is the average amount spent per year for this group of physicians. Gross test dollars per member per year = $159.59.

with a higher utilization as shown by the histograms, which we are beginning to provide at meetings and in newsletters. I sense an interest when the presentation focuses on gains for the customers—namely, the physicians or their patients. A key message is that false-positive test results from unnecessary testing lead to costly and sometimes harmful interventions. These false positives are certainly not value added and detract from one of a physician's most valuable commodities—time (calling the patient, return visits, and so on). Not pursuing abnormal results is a greater malpractice risk than not ordering unwarranted tests.

The educational effort has to be ongoing, data driven, repetitive, and multifaceted. It should include the following:
Graphic presentations
Personalized data feedback
Comparison with peers
Group presentations
Newsletters
One-on-one dialogue

Providing graphic representation personalizes issues for the clinicians and allows them to review their utilization of a particular test.

Cost of Test

Information on the price of tests (or cost) is helpful if provided on an ongoing basis. In the present cost structure, organizations are often paid by the diagnosis-related groups (DRG) or by a capitated fee structure. The cost is more significant than price. Nonetheless, physicians are still interested in the price. In our environment, price, rather than cost, of a test applies to a very small percentage of payers. In the literature, once the price information was no longer published, testing returned to the previous level after 4–6 months. In each case, there had been a temporary decrease in the number of tests ordered during the time when price alerts were provided (84,85). Dresnick and others surveyed a large group of medical students, residents, and faculty and found a common lack of knowledge regarding costs of tests (86). This feedback could be ongoing if physicians were personally using their computers to order. Pricing as well as duplication of tests could be triggered to appear on the monitor simultaneously with the order. Again, good data feedback results in behavior modification, but it must be ongoing.

Thyroid

We have eliminated orders for thyroid profiles, which in the past included a thyroid stimulating hormone (TSH) test, T-4, T-3 uptake, and T-7. We have substituted the TSH, which is more sensitive and specific than the thyroid profile, as the preferred screening test (Fig. 6-13). If it is abnormal, unless specifically ordered as a TSH with no cascade, we automatically report a free T-4 result on the same specimen. All specific orders, such as a thyroxine (T-4) level, continue to be accepted. Only the thyroid profile has been eliminated. However, if a T-7 (a calculation based on a combination of T-4 and T-3 uptake) is ordered, we do a TSH, because we consider this combination a form of thyroid profile. We estimate an annual saving of approximately $70,000 as a result of this change. Prior

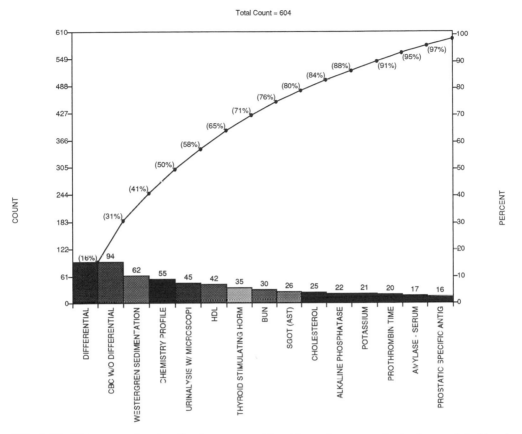

FIG. 6-12. Histogram showing the frequency of the 15 most common tests. A complete blood count with differential is the most common test ordered, and a test for prostatic specific antigen is the fifteenth most common test ordered. The cumulative percentages represented on the line graph demonstrate that these 15 tests represent 97% of the tests ordered.

to making the change the following letter was sent to clinicians, posted in the nursing units, and presented to the medical management committees.

The literature supports using the new, more sensitive TSH assay as the best screening test for hypothyroidism and hyperthyroidism. Approximately 26,000 thyroid profiles with TSH are performed a year by TMCHE/Health Partners Laboratory. One hundred forty-four cases were reviewed. Of these, 70% showed normal thyroid function. TMCHE/HPSA Laboratory will no longer offer a thyroid profile with TSH. If a thyroid profile is ordered, a TSH is performed. If the TSH is abnormal (<0:4, >4.0), then a Free T-4 will be performed. This will provide a significant reduction in cost to the patient and the system without compromising quality or decision making. In order to accommodate those who wish to monitor without a Reflux T-4, we created an order of TSH without Reflux.

Summary: We recommend the use of TSH alone as a screening test in all patients except:

- Those being monitored for thyroid disease.
- Those taking interfering drugs.
- Those suspected to have central hypothyroidism.

Hospitalized patient:

- Stress or acute illness may increase or decrease TSH.
- Dopamine and glucocorticosteroid suppress TSH.

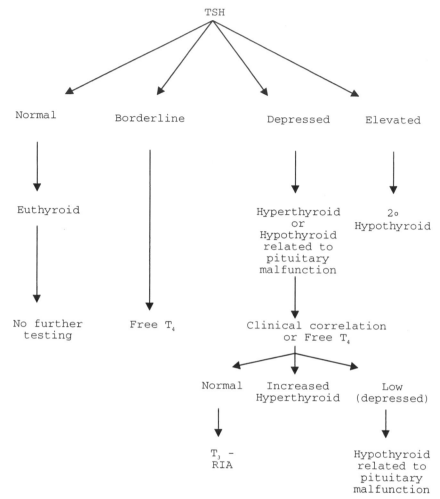

FIG 6-13. Algorithm for thyroid testing (87,88). TSH can be ordered with or without a cascade to free T-4 testing.

We also published an abbreviated form of this letter in our provider newsletter, which was faxed to our high-volume users.

We had been careful to include a large group of respected endocrinologists in the process. We were unsuccessful in getting the physicians into one room. As an alternative, June Clements and I composed a rough draft of the letter and the algorithm that we shared with them, and we discussed it either on the phone or in person with each one. After several drafts we came to a consensus. Once implemented, we met very little resistance from clinicians. The most common call was to question whether or not they could still order the individual tests, which they could. Those few who questioned the wisdom of the change were influenced by the backing of these key endocrinologists. This was a relatively easy cost-saving measure. In retrospect I wonder why we didn't do it earlier. We spent some time reviewing our data to show that this change was worthwhile. It probably would have been sufficient to provide data from the literature. In addition, it improved patient outcome. Frequently T-4 and T-3 are affected by exogenous estrogen with resultant abnormalities that were followed up at additional unwarranted cost and inconvenience to the third-party payers and the patients.

This was an example of a situation in which it would require additional effort for the user to avoid using the process. The TSH would automatically be done with orders for thyroid profiles or T-7s unless the specific tests were ordered. This pattern of implantation favors successful implementation.

LESSONS LEARNED

Initiate discussion with a rough draft of the issue.
Use well-respected champions.
Don't repeat studies well documented in the literature.
For a process change, which positively affects care, use an approach in which it will
    happen automatically unless the clinician does something different.

At the 1-year follow-up, the tests performed changed by the following amounts: TSH had increased by 20%, T-4 had decreased by 65%, T-3 uptake had decreased by 90%, free T-4 had increased by 243%. There were 65% fewer free T-4s than T-4s. (We now do free T-4s in-house; this test was previously sent to a reference lab.) Based on the original number of thyroid profiles, the saving was approximately $40,000 per year.

Reviewing All Tests Greater than $200

All tests costing more than $200 are printed out daily for my review. At times a dialogue with the physician resulted. An example would be chromosome studies to diagnose a rare disease. These tests are best ordered by a pediatric geneticist. In my experience the geneticists sometimes examine the patient and conclude that the previous chromosome study was unwarranted. Many of these related disorders are rare, and a history and physical by an experienced geneticist may be the best screen. The geneticist may request an additional expensive chromosome study. Thus we have two expensive tests rather than one. As a result of these discussions we have encouraged using the geneticist to triage this testing and have decreased chromosome testing.

Some of the expensive tests were groups of tests priced as a profile. I discovered that one of our largest obstetric groups was ordering a urine culture on every prenatal visit. This initiated an examination of the literature followed by a discussion and a change of policy.

The clinical pathway on hepatitis C was also initiated as a result of this review process. The most important part of this process is the dialogue with the individual physicians. This process also serves as a daily reminder to the pathologists to fulfill their role as consultants to the clinicians. By reviewing this list and your monthly sendouts, you can see trends in the utilization of esoteric tests.

Blood Bank

Autologous donations are presently controversial. The cost is equal to or greater than those of allogenic transfusions (blood from individuals of the same species). Autologous blood units are given back to the patient during or after surgery in approximately 50% of all cases. This donation may render a patient anemic, especially if done a few days prior to surgery. The use of hemodilution and cell saver is somewhat less controversial. I have discussed our approach to this in this chapter under the topic of "Preadmission Testing." Data are necessary to change behavior. Any change initiated in a managed-care environment is looked at with suspicion. However, if the blood donations are rendering patients anemic, driving up costs, and not benefiting the patients, we have an obligation to review and try to improve the process.

The blood bank is an area where pathologists have shown leadership in going from whole blood to components, but there remains significant variation in utilization of blood. Some studies that have looked at the appropriateness of blood transfusion in surgical settings suggest that the rate of avoidable transfusions varies between 40% and 60% (89). Transfusions are not given without risk. Although rare, transfusion-transmitted infections and hemolytic transfusion reactions are serious when they occur. The more blood transfusions ordered, the greater the risk of associated morbidity and mortality. Moreover, some of the untoward outcomes of transfusion are not evident immediately. The long-term morbidity costs may be significant expenditures for the health care system. Work-ups for transfusion-related chronic hepatitis may cost several thousand dollars. Interferon used to treat hepatitis C can cost up to $10,000 and still have limited effectiveness (90,91).

To modify behavior related to transfusion decisions, clinicians must be convinced that proposed changes result in better care. This requires medical directors of blood banks to provide scientific data and be available for dialogue with the surgeons and anesthesiologists. This is an area where a change in behavior can have a significant impact. In a study involving 122 general surgeons, orthopedic surgeons, and anesthesiologists, only 31% responded appropriately to questions about transfusion risks and indications (92). Thus education and development of transfusion strategies, including clinical pathways on specific procedures, can improve efficiency of transfusion practices.

For a hospital the aggregate costs of providing blood components represent a large expenditure. Periodic examination of transfusion policies and practices may prove productive in improving the quality of care and potential cost savings. Members of transfusion services of the American Association of Blood Banks now require development and implementation of a quality plan that includes reviewing transfusion-related critical outcomes. The use of recombinant hematopoietic bone-marrow stimulants preoperatively and the potential lowering of the threshold of the hemoglobin required for transfusion are areas of potential cost savings with no adverse impact on patient care. There is a real need for leadership in this area, and we will have to be more creative than merely doing retrospective analysis, which in some studies has been shown to have minimal effect on reducing red blood cell utilization (93).

Hugh Tobin from St. Thomas Hospital in Nashville, Tennessee, studied blood utilization in open-heart surgery. After studying potential variables he concluded that clinical judgment was the key element in making decisions. He provided quality feedback using "low-cost doctor model" (peer comparison). In a 1-year period his hospital experienced a 43% drop in blood and blood-product utilization for open-heart surgery (94).

One-on-one dialogue with strong support from one cardiac surgeon (a champion) has resulted in significant change in the utilization of blood in open-heart surgery at our institution. Cell saver is utilized on all open-heart cases and has made a difference in the usage. It is difficult to quantitate the impact of the cell saver. We initially had standard orders for each open-heart surgery of 10 units of cross-matched blood. Sharing data and continuing the discussion have resulted in the present standing orders of two units of blood cross-matched and two units for type and hold for primary open-heart cases. Redo cases are using either four units cross-matched and four units on hold or four units cross-matched and two units on hold. Fresh-frozen plasma usage had gone from four units routinely ordered to none. The fresh-frozen plasma is now ordered on an as-needed basis and is only requested occasionally. When possible, platelets are given from a single donor source and utilized in less than 50% of the cases. At one time, six units of platelets were standard with all open-heart surgery. This change has occurred as a result of shared data, peer comparison, and continuous dialogue. This did not happen overnight. Some physicians adapted to change readily; others resisted it. Both play a role in change. Those who resist, demand more data and protect the status quo, which serves to fine-tune our processes. To modify behavior successfully, we need to recognize the different roles clinicians play in change and their individual needs. The most important data come from those who adopt changes early and share their successful outcomes with others.

LESSONS LEARNED

Feedback and a champion who utilizes data and presents variation studies are essential.
Keep it simple by focusing on one DRG.
Peer comparison is a powerful tool.

Other Measures to Improve Efficiency and Effectiveness in the Lab

Microbiology

The following are some ways in which microbiology can help improve processes in the lab:

1. Eliminate Gram's stains as routine on cervical vaginal cultures. They are not reliable for diagnosis.
2. Realize that DNA probes for gonococcus and chlamydia are more dependable than cultures. There are fewer false-negative cultures because of temperature or timing during culture transportation when using DNA probes.
3. Avoid work-up of spinal fluids if chemistry and cell counts are normal. (We had previously done cultures routinely on all spinal fluids, including those from myelograms.)
4. Do not repeat *Clostridium difficile* testing within 1 week of prior examination. All patients should have copious diarrhea and antibiotic usage within 30 days of any testing (95).
5. Monitor single blood cultures. Sensitivity and diagnostic reliability are increased by collecting two or three specimens. Multiple specimens help differentiate transient, intermittent, and contiguous bacteremia and help to distinguish true bacteremia from contaminated blood cultures. This is true both for adults and for infants and neonates (96). It has also been shown that routine blood cultures for fever in the preoperative period are not cost-effective (97).
6. Eliminate blood culture contamination by paying attention to details of blood collection and providing feedback to those performing the procedure. The cost of a single

contaminated culture can be as high as $4,000 (98). By publishing our data and giving one-on-one instruction to those involved with a contaminated culture, we have reduced our contamination rate by 75%. Our goal is less than 2% contamination rate for blood cultures. Our experience shows a higher contamination rate when patient-care technicians or nurses draw blood than when phlebotomists draw it. With time, continued dialogue, and training, the data for patient-care technicians and contaminated blood cultures have improved dramatically.

7. Avoid stool testing for *Shigella, Salmonella,* and *Campylobacter,* as well as ova and parasites, 48 hours after hospitalization.
8. Eliminate fecal Gram's stains for neutrophils. In our experience, they are unreliable as a basis for performing a stool culture or patient management.

Chemistry

Discuss tests to be used for screening in the outpatient setting. Our goal is development of smaller profiles used to screen nonsymptomatic patients, most of whom are seen as part of an annual physical examination. Medicare is presently defining specific profiles that will be reimbursed, and other third-party payers are likely to follow this pattern. Eliminate lactic dehydrogenase (LDH) isoenzymes unless approved by a pathologist. (This should be very rare, if ever.)

Histology

1. Examine only placentas with history of clinical abnormalities.
2. Review variation in utilization of special studies. For example, trichrome and iron stains on all liver biopsies before the standard hematoxylin and eosin (H&E) sections are reviewed for the presence or absence of pathology. Focus on any standard usage occurring before review of the routine H&E slides.
3. Increase utilization of standardized reporting formats. Standardized reporting consistently results in a more complete report. Once the physicians are familiar with the format, they can readily identify the location of data that they consider critical.

SUMMARY

Implementation of appropriate test utilization requires leadership and passion combined with a plan.

- Leadership skills to encourage, and at times insist on, participation and creativity, with significant action follow-up. Leaders would do well to know how to elicit creativity. If you can think, you can be creative.
- **Effective** leaders clarify what to achieve and can coach on "how to achieve."
- **Passion** for the work is extremely important. Passion is contagious, and it is not only important to you but good for the system.
- You must have a **plan**, which includes sound innovations, priorities, and **commitment**.
- **Quality** is a way of life, not an intermittent stop. We must eliminate waste, whether it is part of a process or an entire process. If it doesn't contribute value, eliminate it.

Our challenge is not just to cut costs but to improve the quality of care. More is not better. Unnecessary tests increase waste.

The commitment to eliminating waste must include believing that your efforts make a difference; making time to observe for variation; obtaining input from all levels; supporting positive change; being willing to follow up tenaciously; understanding that there may not be immediate or 100% acceptance; and measuring to show improvement.

Poor quality costs. But if you attempt to improve appropriateness, you should fasten your seatbelt. It may be a rough ride.

REFERENCES

1. Danzon PM, Manning WG, Marquis MS: Factors affecting laboratory test use and prices. *Health Care Financing Rev* 1984;5:23–24.
2. Davies N, Felder LH: Applying brakes to the runaway American health care system. *JAMA* 1990;63:73–76.
3. Eisenberg JM, Esenkey VW: Cost containment and changing physicians practice behavior. *JAMA* 1981;246:2195–2201.
4. Woolf SH, Kamerow DB: Testing for uncommon conditions. The heroic search for positive test results. *Arch Intern Med* 1990;150(12):2451–2458.
5. Tierney WJ, Miller ME, McDonald CJ: The effect on test ordering of informing physicians of the charges for outpatient diagnostic tests. *N Engl J Med* 1990;322(21):1499–1504.
6. Bushick JB, Eisenberg JM, Kinman J, Cebul RD, Schwartz JS: Pursuit of abnormal coagulation screening tests generates hidden pre-operative costs. *J Gen Intern Med* 1989;4:493–497.
7. Winkelman JW: Less utilization of the clinical laboratory produces disproportionately small true cost reduction. *Hum Pathol* 1984;15:499–501.
8. Califano J: Health care misplaces millions, excerpt from *The New York Times*. Published in *The Arizona Daily Star*, April 16, 1989, p. C-1.
9. Albertson D: Lab tests cited in the high cost of defensive medicine. *MLO* 1993;25:17–18.
10. Macario A, Rizen MF, Thisted RA, Kim S, Ordkin FK, Phelps C: Reassessment of preoperative laboratory testing has changed the test-ordering patterns of physicians. *Surg Gynecol Obstet* 1992;175:539–547.
11. Summerlon N: Positive and negative factors in defensive medicine: a questionable study of general practitioners. *BMJ* 1995;310:27–29.
12. Fitzgibbon RJ. Three fourths of physicians overtest due to malpractice threat. *MLO* 1989;21:9.
13. Woodward C, Rosser WW: A national survey of the impact of medico-legal liability on patterns of practice. *Can Med Assoc J* 1989;141:291–299.
14. Link K, Centor R, Buchsbaum D, Witherspoon J: Why physicians don't pursue abnormal laboratory tests. *Hum Pathol* 1984;15:75–78.
15. Griner PF, Glaser RJ: Misuse of laboratory test and diagnostic procedures. *N Engl J Med* 1982;307:1336–1337.
16. Chapman B: Reducing lab tests use. *CAP Today*, 1995;9(6):20, 22, 24, 26.
17. Tierney WM, Miller MG, McDonald CJ: The effect on test ordering of informing physicians of the charges of diagnostic testing. *N Engl J Med* 1990;322(21):1499.
18. Billing J, Eddy D: Physician decision making limited by medical evidence. *Business and Health*, November 1987, pp. 23–28.
19. Johnson H Jr, Knee-loli S, Butler TA, Munoz E, Wise L: Are routine preoperative laboratory screening tests necessary to evaluate ambulatory surgical patients? *Surgery* 1988;104(4):639–645.
20. Narr BJ, Hansen TR, Warner MA: Preoperative laboratory screening in healthy Mayo patients: cost-effective elimination of tests and unchanged outcomes. *Mayo Clin Proc* 1991;66(2):155–159.
21. Gewirtz A, Miller M, Keys T: The clinical usefulness of the pre-operative bleeding time. *Arch Pathol Lab Med* 1996;120:353–356.
22. Bachmann F: Diagnostic approach to mild bleeding disorders. *Semin Hematol* 1980;17:292–305.
23. Hougie C: Hemophilia and related conditions-congenital deficiencies of prothrombin (factor II), factor V, and factors VII to XII, In: Williams WJ, Beutler E, Erslev AJ, Lichtman MA, eds., *Hematology*, 3rd ed. New York: McGraw-Hill, 1983, pp. 1381–1399.
24. Eisenberg JM, Clarke JR, Sussman SA: Prothrombin and partial thromboplastin time as preoperative screening tests. *Arch Surg* 1982;117:48–51.
25. Robbins JA, Rose SD: Partial thromboplastin time as a screening test. *Ann Intern Med* 1979;90:796–797.
26. Kaplan EB, Sheiner LB, Boeckmann AJ, et al: The usefulness of preoperative laboratory screening. *JAMA* 1985;253(24):3576–3581.
27. Turnbull JM, Buck C: The value of preoperative screening investigations in otherwise healthy individuals. *Arch Intern Med* 1987;147:1101–1105.
28. Suchman AL, Griner PF: Diagnostic uses of the activated partial thromboplastin time and prothrombin time. *Ann Intern Med* 1986;104(6):810–816.

29. Durbridge TC, Edwards F, Edwards RG, Atkinson M: Evaluation of benefits of screening tests done immediately on admission to the hospital. *Clin Chem* 1976;22:968–971.
30. Korvin CC, Pearce RH, Stanley J: Admissions screening: clinical benefits. *Ann Intern Med* 1975;83(2):197–203.
31. Boland BJ, Wollan PC, Silverstein MD: Yield of laboratory tests for case finding in ambulatory general medical examination. *Am J Med* 1996;101(2):142–152.
32. Ruttimann S, Clemencon D, Dubach UC: Usefulness of complete blood counts as a case finding in medical out-patients. *Ann Intern Med* 1993;116:44–50.
33. Valenstein P, Schifman RB: Duplicate laboratory order. *Arch Pathol Lab Med* 1996;120:917–921.
34. Schoenenberger RA, Milenko J, Tanasijevic MD, Ashish JH, Bates DW: Appropriateness of antiepileptic drug level monitoring. *JAMA* 1995;274:1622–1626.
35. Burke MD: Laboratory tests: basic concepts and realistic expectations. *Postgrad Med* 1978;63(4):53–55, 58, 60.
36. Chapman B: Striking the right balance with TDMs. *CAP Today* 1996;10:1, 24–34.
37. Mason CD, Winter ME: Appropriateness of sampling times for therapeutic drug monitoring. *Am J Hosp Pharm* 1984;41:1796–801.
38. Bussey H, Hoffman EW: A prospective evaluation of therapeutic drug monitoring. *Therapeut Drug Monit* 1983;5:245–8.
39. Levine, M, McCollon, Chang T, Orr J: Evaluation of serum phenytoin monitoring in an acute care setting. *Ther Drug Monit* 1988;10:50–57.
40. Wong PKH, Brown DL, Bachmann KA, Forney, RB, Hicks CI, Schwartz JI: Optimal dosing of phenytoin: an evaluation of the timing and appropriateness of serum level monitoring. *Hosp Formul* 1989;24:219–223.
41. Mennemeyer ST, Winkelman JW: Searching for inaccuracy in clinical laboratory testing using Medicare data: evidence for prothrombin time. *JAMA* 1993;269:1030–1033.
42. Wilt VM, Gums JG, Ahmed OI, Moore LM: Outcome analysis of a pharmacist-managed anticoagulation service. *Pharmacotherapy* 1995;15(6):732–739.
43. Lee YP, Schommer JC: Effects of a pharmacist-managed anticoagulation clinic on warfarin-related hospital readmissions. *Am J Health-Syst Pharm* 1996;53:1581–2.
44. Radley AS, Hall J: The establishment and evaluation of a pharmacist-developed anticoagulant clinic. *Pharm J* 1994;252:91–92.
45. Wilson Norton JL, Gibson DL: Establishing an outpatient anticoagulant clinic in a community hospital. *Am J Health-Syst Pharm* 1995;53:1151–1157.
46. Engle JP: Anticoagulation: practice focus in an ambulatory clinic. *J Pharm Pract* 1990;3(5):329–357.
47. Merryfield DW, Ayers TG, Wilkson CA, Williams RB: Clinical pharmacy services in a rehabilitation facility. *Am J Hosp Pharm* 1983;40:1529–1532.
48. Charney R, Leddormado E, Rose DN, Fuster V: Anticoagulation clinics and the monitoring of anticoagulant therapy. *Int J Cardiol* 1988;18:197–206.
49. Ellis RF, Stephens MA, Sharp GB: Evaluation of a pharmacy-managed warfarin-monitoring service to coordinate inpatient and outpatient therapy. *Am J Hosp Pharm* 1992;49:387–394.
50. Macgregor SH, Hamley JG, Dunbar JA, Dodd TR, Cromarty JA: Evaluation of primary care anticoagulant clinic managed by a pharmacist. *BMJ* 1996;312(7060):560.
51. Evans WE, Schentag JJ, Jusko WJ: *Applied pharmacokinetics: principles of therapeutic drug monitoring*, 3rd ed. Spokane: Applied Therapeutics, Inc.,1992, pp. 31–32.
52. Ansell JE, Buttaro ML, Thomas OV, et al: Consensus guidelines for coordinated outpatient oral anticoagulation therapy management. *Ann Pharmacother* 1997;31:604–615.
53. Klepser ME, Herbert J: Evaluation of a systemic warfarin: dosing protocol. *P & T* 1994;866–876.
54. Gurwitz JH, Avorn J, Ross-Degnan D, Choodnovsky I, Ansell J: Aging and the anticoagulant response to warfarin therapy. *Ann Intern Med* 1992;116(11):901–904.
55. Wynne H, Cope L, Kelly P, Whittingham T, Edwards C, Kamali F: The influence of age, liver size and enantiomer concentrations on warfarin requirements. *Br J Clin Pharm* 1995;40(3):203–207.
56. Fihn SD, Callahan CM, Martin DC, McDonell MB, Henikoff JG, White RH: The risk for and severity of bleeding complications in elderly patients treated with warfarin. *Ann Intern Med* 1996;124(11):970–979.
57. Coumadin package insert. DuPont Pharmaceuticals, 1995.
58. Harrison L, Johnston M, Massicotte MP, Crowther M, Moffat K, Hirsh J: Comparison of 5-mg and 10-mg loading doses in initiation of warfarin therapy. *Ann Intern Med* 1997;126(2):133–136.
59. Rivey MP, Wood RD, Allington DR, Stratton TP, Erickson CC, Stenson TA: Pharmacy-managed protocol for warfarin use in orthopedic surgery patients. *Am J Health-Syst Pharm* 1995;52(12):1310–1316.
60. Bridgen ML: Oral anticoagulation therapy. *Postgrad Med* 1996;99(6):81–100.
61. Onderdonk AB, Winkelman JW, Orni-Wasserlau RO: Eliminating unnecessary urine cultures to reduce costs. *Lab Med* 1996;27:829–832.
62. Murray PR, Baron EJ, Pfaller MA, Penover FC, Yolken RH: *Manual of clinical microbiology,* 6th ed., Washington, D.C.: ASM Press 1995, p. 309.
63. US Preventative Services Task Force, Screening for Cervical Cancer: *Guide to clinical preventive services: an assessment of the effectiveness of 169 interventions.* Baltimore: Williams and Wilkins, 1989, pp. 57–62.
64. ACOG Technical Bulletin: Cervical cytology: evaluation and management of abnormalities, #183, Aug 1993.
65. No author: Florida hospital cuts utilization by reducing standing orders. Medicare publication, Dec 1989;17:5–7.
66. Studnicki J, Bradham DD, Mashburn J, Foulis PR, Straumford JV: Measuring the impact of standing orders on lab utilization. *Lab Med* 1992;23:24–28.

67. Fan K, Morris AJ, Roller LB: Application of rejection criteria for bacterial enteric pathogens. *J Clin Microbiol* 1993;31:2233.

68. Koontz F, Weinstock JV: The approach to stool examination for parasites. *Gastroenterol Clin North Am* 1996;25(3):435–449.

69. Brook RH: Practice guidelines and practicing medicine. *JAMA* 1989;262:3027–3030.

70. Woolf SH: Practice guidelines, a new reality in medicine. *Arch Intern Med* 1990;150:1811–1818.

71. Nelson EC, Mohr JJ, Batalden PB, Plume SK: Improving health care, part I: the clinical value compass. *J Qual Improv* 1996;22:243–256.

72. Clark M: Parameters project "biggest ever." *CAP Today* 1990;4:1, 13–15.

73. Schaldach DE: Measuring quality and cost of care: evaluation of an amputation clinical pathway. *J Vasc NURS* 1997;15:13–20.

74. Andersson S: Scripps health: quality planning for clinical processes of care. *Qual Lett Healthc Lead* 1993;5:2–4.

75. Nelson CE, Mohr JJ, Batalden PB, Plums SK: Improving healthcare, part 1: the clinical value compass. *J Qual Improv* 1996;22:243–258.

76. O'Malley S: Getting physician buy-in to standardization efforts. *Qual Lett Healthc Lead* 1997;9.2–11.

77. Weiland O, Chen M, Lindh G, Mattsson L, et al. Efficacy of human leucocyte alpha-interferon treatment for chronic hepatitis C virus infect. [Corrected and republished with original paging. Article originally printed in *Scand J Infect Dis* 1995;27(4):319–324.]

78. Dixon RH, Lazio J: Utilization of clinical chemistry services by medical house staff: an analysis. *JAMA* 1974;134:1064–1069.

79. Wachtel TJ, O'Sullivan P: Practice guidelines to reduce testing in the hospital. *Gen Intern Med* 1990,5:335–341.

80. Studnicki J, Stevens C, Knisely L: A feedback system for reducing excessive laboratory tests. *Arch Pathol Lab Med* 1993;117:35–39.

81. Beck JR: Does feedback reduce inappropriate test ordering. *Arch Pathol Lab Med* 1993;117:33–34.

82. Kroenke K, Hanley JF, Copley JB, Matthews JI, Davis CE, Foulks CJ: Improving house staff ordering of three common laboratory tests. Reductions in test ordering need not result in under utilization. *Med Care* 1987;25(10):928–935.

83. Dowling PT, Alfonsi G, Brown MI, Culpepper L: An education program to reduce unnecessary laboratory rests by residents. *Acad Med* 1989;64:410–412.

84. Tierney WM, Miller ME, McDonald CJ: The effect on test ordering of informing physicians of the charges for outpatient diagnostic tests. *N Engl J Med* 1990;322:1499–1504.

85. Eisenberg JM, Sankey VW: Cost containment and changing physicians' practice behavior. *JAMA* 1981;246:2195–2201.

86. Dresnick SJ, Roth WI, Linn BS, Prat TC, Blum A: The physician's role in the cost containment model. *JAMA* 1979;241:1606–1609.

87. Feldkamp CS, Carey JL: An algorithmic approach to thyroid function testing in a managed care setting. *Am J Clin Pathol* 1996;105:11–16.

88. Davey RX, Clark MI, Webster AR: Assessment of an algorithm for thyroid function testing based on initial TSH measurement. *Med J Aust* 1996;164(6):329–332.

89. Audet A: Red blood cell transfusion in patients undergoing orthopedic surgery: a HCFA quality improvement project (HCQIP). *Eye Improv* 1996;111(24):4–6.

90. Dusheiko GM, Roberts JA: Treatment of chronic type B and C hepatitis with interferon alfa: an economic approach. *Hepatology* 1995;22:1863–1873.

91. Salem-Schatz SR, Avorn J, Soumerai SB: Influence of clinical knowledge, organizational context, and practice style on transfusion decision making. *JAMA* 1990;264:471–475.

92. AuBuchan JP: Blood transfusion options: improving outcomes and reducing costs. *Arch Pathol Lab Med* 1997;121:4–47.

93. Lam HTC, Schweitzer SO, Petz L, et al: Are retrospective peer-review transfusion monitoring systems effective in reducing red blood cell utilization. *Arch Pathol Lab Med* 1996;120(9):810–816.

94. Paxton A: In Nashville hospital, drop in blood usage is dramatic. *CAP Today* 1996;10:72–73.

95. Katz DA, Lynch ME, Littenerg B: Clinical prediction rules to optimize cytoxin testing for *Clostridium difficile* in hospitalized patients with diarrhea. *Am J Med* 1996;100:487–495.

96. Schifman RB, Bachner P, Howanitz PJ: Blood culture quality improvement. *Arch Pathol Lab Med* 1996;120:999–1002.

97. Theyer CP, Bangard FS, Klein SR: Are blood cultures effective in the evaluation of fever in perioperative patients? *Am J Surg* 1991;162:615–619.

98. Bates DW, Lee G, Goldman L, Lee TH: Contaminant blood cultures and resource utilization: the true consequence of false positive results. *JAMA* 1991;265(3):365–369.

7

Clinical Laboratory Automation: Concepts and Directions

Rodney S. Markin

Clinical laboratory automation has evolved over the last 15 years from a concept to a reality. The first steps in clinical laboratory automation were to replicate or emulate the function of the human in the clinical laboratory. The first systems were implemented in clinical laboratories in Japan (1–6). Their operation was a significant step toward overcoming the fears of implementing automation in the health care environment.

North America and Western Europe have lagged far behind Japan in creating and implementing clinical laboratory automation. At first glance, the hindrance appears to be related to two issues: lack of financial incentive to invest in automation and lack of understanding of the principles of automation.

Historically, we have enjoyed significant revenue streams and profits from the clinical laboratory. So why would we invest in an emerging technology such as clinical laboratory automation? We have no perceived financial incentive to do so. In the current environment, the profits are slim and the costs are relatively high compared with our historical prospective. Investing in new technologies, such as automation, makes potential buyers nervous. At this point in the history of clinical laboratory automation, the costs are somewhat high, ranging in price from $1 to $5 million. The laboratory community wants proven technology without risk and a "competitive" pricing structure. Most do not believe that clinical laboratory automation functions adequately, even though they may not recognize "functionality" when it is presented to them. The ability to drive down costs will be related in part to clinical laboratories that exhibit some risk-taking behavior or are early adopters of technology, stepping to the forefront to embrace clinical laboratory automation. Investing in advanced technology will help drive down costs and move up production schedules.

The purpose of this chapter is to provide a starting point for those interested in learning about clinical laboratory automation and its potential.

THE PRODUCT OF THE CLINICAL LABORATORY (AND EXTRACTION TOOLS)

The product of the clinical laboratory is information. Our product information is extracted from biological samples, including serum, plasma, spinal fluid, whole blood, other body fluids, tissues, and cytology specimens. Historically, the clinical laboratory has thought of itself as an operation that has both responded to requests for results and provided results. It is clear in the retrospective analysis that our business is providing information, and in fact, approximately 50% of the component information in computerized patient records (CPR) is provided by the clinical laboratory (Fig. 7-1).

Clinical laboratory automation will occur for several reasons, the first of which is its ability to improve laboratory operations. At the forefront of laboratory operation im-

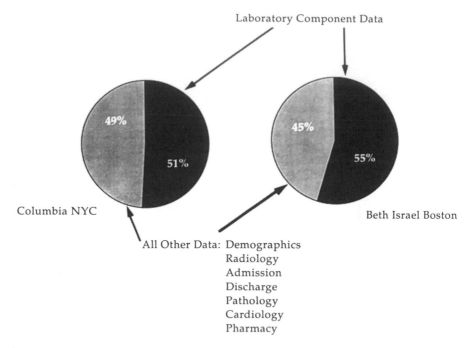

FIG. 7-1. Chart showing the relative amount of component data composing the computerized patient record (CPR). The laboratory data provide for greater than 50% of this clinical laboratory information. (Data from Enterprise Analysis Corporation.)

provement is cost savings. We are being required to reduce the cost of providing the information we extract from biological samples. The information that we provide has now become a commodity, as opposed to the historical "cottage industry" approach to clinical laboratories and the captive client base.

Tools to improve clinical laboratory operations include the following: (a) information systems, such as the currently installed base of laboratory information systems (LIS); (b) automation technology, which includes software for automation; (c) robotics; (d) enhancements to clinical laboratory instruments and point-of-care testing; (e) identification technologies, such as bar codes or other, more sophisticated methodologies such as digital read/write tags; and (f) transportation systems, including those operated by people, automated guided vehicles (AGV mobile robots), and a variety of "conveyorlike" transportation systems from the current clinical laboratory automation vendors.

PATIENT AND PROGRAM ISSUES

The most important factors affecting laboratory operations are the following:

Patient demands
Declining reimbursement
Special programs that implement advanced technologies
The drive to develop utilization management schemes and outcomes improvements

Patient demands are being driven by the speed with which our society moves and the perceived relationship between quality and timeliness of service. We are all facing declines in reimbursement as evidenced by changes to the bottom line of clinical laboratory operations and the decisions to sell off or spin off laboratory operations from larger organizations (e.g., the extraction of Corning Clinical Labs from the Corning Family to form Quest Laboratories).

Special programs that involve the application of sophisticated technology—such as solid organ transplantation, bone marrow transplantation, chemotherapy, and other related entities—require information from the clinical laboratory that is beyond the usual requirements driven by the general practice of medicine (7). Immunoassays for immunosuppressive agents such as cyclosporine (Neoral, Novartis Pharmaceuticals, East Hanover, New Jersey), FK506 (Fujisawa USA, Deerfield, Illinois), and mycophenolate mofetil (Roche Pharmaceuticals, Palo Alto, California), as well as tissue typing and other rapid-response requirements, are critical for the implementation and operation of a high-technology program. The programs detract from the bottom line of the laboratory operation, even though they add to the bottom line of the enterprise (where the clinical laboratory is a part of the enterprise).

UTILIZATION MANAGEMENT AND OUTCOMES

Utilization management and patient outcomes have become important topics in the past several years. *Utilization management* is a term that is applied to all facets of health care delivery. It implies a mechanism for management of resources at the level of the individual provider and beyond. Utilization management responsibilities have been introduced into the clinical laboratory without a sufficient mechanism to implement such schemes. Information systems–driven clinical laboratory automation solutions will provide a mechanism for implementing utilization management algorithms and rules-based testing.

The ability of the laboratory to enable real-time utilization management algorithms will change the face of health care delivery as we know it. The term *outcomes* is frequently used in medical and clinical laboratory discussions. The outcome being discussed, of course, is that of the patient. We should ask, "How did the patient fare as he moved through the health care process?"

One of the problems we face in applying knowledge to improve outcomes is a lack of understanding of the natural history of disease processes. We need to relate outcomes to the natural history of a disease process and then plot factors that positively or negatively influence the patient against that natural history. At this point we have few good or reasonable tools with which to measure outcomes. There is the currently accepted technique of the "wallet biopsy" to determine how the patient's wallet did as we moved the patient and his or her wallet through the process of health care delivery. The wallet biopsy does not tell the entire story and is not a reflection of your medical care or your health. As we move forward in improving the process of health care delivery, the need for clinical laboratory automation will become apparent.

DEVELOPMENT OF CLINICAL LABORATORY AUTOMATION

In developing clinical laboratory automation, the focus of development can move in two directions: the technology (8–12) or the patient (13–16).

A focus on technology would define the important issues in the clinical laboratory and require the patient to "revolve" around the requirements of the laboratory. A focus on the patient provides an automation solution that will serve the needs of the patients and be useful to those who work in the laboratory.

A number of issues and factors must be taken into account when designing a software-driven automation solution. As we develop the architecture for automation systems, it is clear that we should start from our 5–10-year horizon, with respect to the expected state of health care delivery, and work backward to develop flexible architectural platforms. This leads us to the premise that the health care delivery system database or integrated delivery (IDS) database is actually based upon the collection, analysis, and application of data and information from patients, individually and collectively with different types of diseases or disorders. The database can be used to define the factors affecting patient outcomes and develop protocols, pathways, or processes to deliver health care. When taking an architectural structure into account, it is very important to look at the information necessary to deliver care adequately to the patient. A distinction between on-site and off-site testing operations as applied to individual tests, patient location, and service level requirements must be evaluated. To develop our approach, we took into account the relative use of the information with respect to the patient's disease or disorder and the patient's location. It is clear that certain tests are necessary for rapid diagnosis and treatment of the patient. Those tests are most likely to be performed on currently "automated" analyzers or instruments and to be done near the patient.

It is also clear that this necessity has driven the development of near-patient testing. The profiles or tests that are available on near-patient testing technologies are useful in diagnosis and treatment and may play a part in influencing the outcome of the patient through the relative availability of the information they provide. From an architectural standpoint, it is clear that the ability to physically segregate on-site and off-site tests is important. The relationship of the information needs to be understood so that information from an on-site test can be used to direct testing algorithms that may influence the off-site test.

RELATIONSHIPS BETWEEN TESTING AND OUTCOMES

As discussed earlier in this chapter, outcomes relate to the natural history of disease. The concept of the natural history of disease is a fundamental one in pathology and is often overlooked. The real issues of patient management and outcomes have their foundation in this simple thought. The natural history is a long-term issue that may be divided into small segments or episodes, such as an episode of care. The outcome from an episode of care may or may not influence the outcome of the natural history of a disease, depending upon the specific outcome of the episode of care and its relationship to the natural history of disease or disorder. Most people think in terms of short-term issues and hence short-term outcomes, but the most important issues involve long-term outcome and general issues of health. If we analyze medical literature in general, it is very clear that long-term outcomes have been the important focus in diabetic care, diagnosis and treatment of cancer, transplantation, corrective surgery for congenital defects, and many other ailments. There is a distinct relationship between therapy and outcome or treatment, and outcome that has been well defined, especially in the cancer treatment literature.

There is also a distinct relationship between laboratory results and outcomes. These relationships have not been well defined. However, anyone having practiced medicine should support the notion that the relationships in general are clear. Examples brought forth in the past have been the number of electrolyte determinations performed in a given time frame for patients who are on intravenous therapy versus those not on intravenous therapy. As long as your kidneys are functioning adequately and you don't have any major fluid losses (e.g., diarrhea), are not on diuretic therapy, or do not have an inherited metabolic electrolyte disorder (e.g., Conn's syndrome), sequential electrolyte determinations are unnecessary. Moreover, it is common knowledge that mammals are not electrically charged. It therefore makes sense that in the absence of some large-volume loss, passive ion determinations such as chloride assays are unnecessary.

HEALTH CARE DELIVERY SYSTEM DATABASES AND INFORMATION

The concept of the community health information network has been discussed in the medical and information system technology community for the last 5–7 years (Fig. 7-2). As information technology improves by quantum leaps, the implementation of a community health information network or integrated delivery system network is possible. The integrated delivery system network would tie together multiple provider entities, including hospitals, laboratories, pharmacies, physicians' offices, insurance companies, banks, and employers (payers). The relative access to this information would be and should be security restricted. The important point is that there would be a common repository for clinical information that would remain available over time.

One of the significant drawbacks to the development of integrated delivery system networks is the relative lack of standardization of the clinical laboratory and medical lexicons. Several groups have worked on codification schemes so that the descriptions of patients, their symptoms and clinical signs, therapy, laboratory results, radiology results, and other information could be codified uniformly.

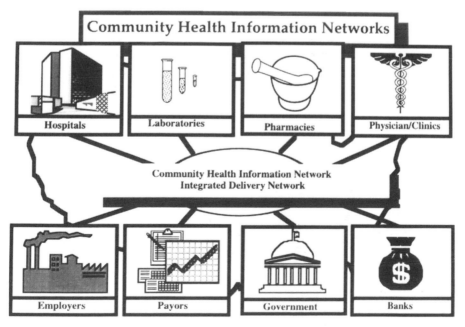

FIG. 7-2. Diagram of the community health information network (CHIN). The CHIN or integrated delivery network (IDN) ties together information from health care providers, employers, banks, and payers.

One of the significant issues that we have encountered as we have dealt with integrated delivery system networks and how laboratories will fit into the flow of information is the lack of uniformity in the information delivered by multiple clinical laboratories (Table 7-1). This lack of uniformity is a result of using different instruments with different methodologies that usually have different reference ranges. From a practical perspective, results from different methodologies cannot be plotted on the same graph because of a lack of a defined relationship between the results from different methods. If these data cannot be graphed on the same axis, then the results cannot be used by an algorithm to determine whether a result may spawn an additional test or tests, or be used to cancel a test or make a clinical decision.

There are two possible approaches with respect to the usability of results. The first would be to standardize the clinical laboratory instrumentation. In other words, we need to define one common chemistry instrument with a set of defined methodologies, one common hematology instrument with a set of defined methodologies, one common immunoassay instrument with a set of defined methodologies, and so forth. This seems somewhat impractical because a large number of *in vitro* diagnostics manufacturers (IVD manufacturers) have viable products and services. The choices would be difficult.

The second approach would be to implement the normalization of algorithms to interrelate the data from different instruments using different methodologies. This is the approach we have taken to develop the first level of the data normalization technologies. The development of technology to normalize clinical laboratory results is complex. We are currently compiling statistical information to define all the different methodologies currently available in the clinical laboratory and some retrospective methodologies.

Several attempts have been made to develop a naming scheme or classification scheme for clinical laboratory results and other medical nomenclature systems. The most notable is the LONIC from Clem McDonald's group at the Reagenstrief Hospital (17). This scheme provides method-based naming or nomenclature for clinical laboratory tests.

One of the potential applications of the integrated delivery network database is the ability to allow multiple institutions to communicate. The possibility exists of having multiple laboratory automation systems (LAS) in different-sized laboratories, all of which would communicate demographic data and other clinically relevant information about patients via the community health information network (Fig. 7-3). Patient speci-

TABLE 7-1. *Selected results by analyte from 1996 CAP chemistry and ligand assay survey data*

Test name	Sample	No. of methods	Range of survey result means (X)
Cholesterol*	LP-01	35	234.7–295.2
Acid phosphatase	C-01	10	1.34–6.60
Alkaline phosphatase	C-02	32	226.8–375.5
Creatine kinase	IE-01	19	300.0–397.2
Creatine kinase-MB fraction	IE-03	10	39.0–84.0
Carcinoembryonic antigen (CEA)	K-02	11	22.49–39.68
Human chorionic Gonadotropin (HCG)	K-02	20	78.99–133.35
Estradiol	Y-01	16	851.00–1755.95

These data represent an extract from a College of American Pathologists (CAP) *Check Sample* report published in 1996 with data from the year 1996 (for original data please contact either the CAP or LAB-InterLink, Inc. approximately 250 pages).

*Cholesterol measurements have been the focus of standardization during the last 5 years as a part of the National Cholesterol Education Program (NCEP).

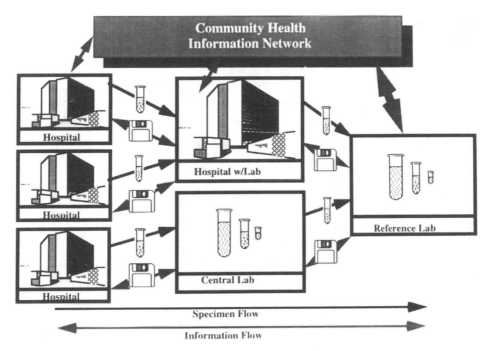

FIG. 7-3. Multiple clinical laboratories spread across the wide geographic distance connected electronically through the CHIN sharing information that may be related to laboratory specimens.

mens would be tested at various locations, depending upon the clinical necessity of the test, the economy of scale, and other operational factors affecting the laboratory or the delivery network. The specimens would be interchanged between laboratories. Specimens would contain the appropriate identification and clinical information necessary to carry out algorithmic testing at one level in the peripheral testing sites such as community hospitals, at the second level at the core laboratory or regional laboratory level, and at a third level for the reference laboratory. In all these situations, the same or different algorithms could be used. The important issue is the transmission of clinical lab results—along with the appropriate patient identifier—either with the specimen or through the integrated delivery system network, or both.

LABORATORY OPERATIONS

Laboratory operations are divided into multiple subsets. The most important laboratory operations issues are physical layout, flow of specimens, and the way the flow of specimens relates to the flow of information (13).

The traditional flow of specimens through the clinical laboratory is related to the organizational structure of testing and the fact that most people operate in a batch mode. We tend to batch our meals, our learning, our work, and other types of processes. We have therefore constructed a laboratory operation with defined cut-offs for accumulation of specimens or inclusion of a specimen into a testing batch. We have also adopted the use of aliquots so that multiple parallel specimens can be sent to laboratories for parallel batch testing. This traditional approach has worked for the past 50–60 years (Fig. 7-4).

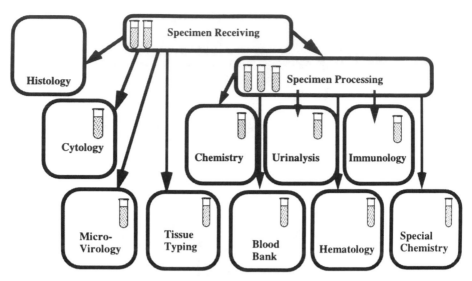

FIG. 7-4. Schematic diagram of a traditional laboratory layout based upon "classic" laboratory sections and batch analysis.

Two additional approaches may be used for organizing laboratory testing and the flow of specimens. The first is an assembly line–like process called a product line. In this case, the product line could be related to the matrix. In a laboratory with some 500 potential tests on the menu, a product line for each test type would be impractical. A product line approach using a matrix is much more realistic, as the two proposed matrixes would be specimens with cells and specimens without cells (e.g., serum, plasma, centrifuged fluids). Laboratory organization would be based on a series of concentric circles or areas that contain different levels of automated technology (Fig. 7-5). Central receiving or

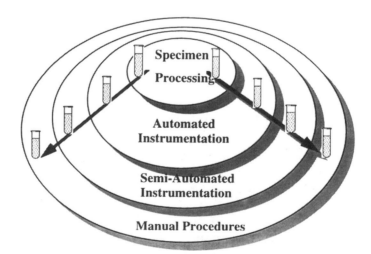

FIG. 7-5. Schematic diagram of a clinical laboratory layout based on product line. One product line would transport specimens that contain cells. The other product line would transport specimens that are centrifuged (acellular, serum, or plasma).

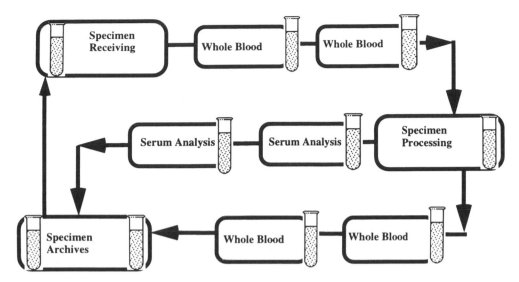

FIG. 7-6. A schematic diagram of a serial specimen processing line which moves each specimen on a network of transportation to logical devices where specimen processing or analysis may occur.

specimen receiving and specimen processing would be located in the center-most concentric circle. The next outward ring would be automated technology and would include chemistry, immunoassay, hematology, coagulation, and potentially, urinalysis. Semiautomated technology would be located in the next concentric circle. Manual procedures—such as evaluation of peripheral smears, cytology, and so on—would be performed in the outermost concentric circle.

We are trying to achieve a serial analysis approach to laboratory operations (Fig. 7-6). The serial analysis approach was chosen because it facilitates the concept of the tube or specimen representing the patient. The concept is simply to give the patient's specimen access to all diagnostic or analytical modalities and locations in the clinical laboratory, just as the patient has access to different parts of the health care delivery system. By having random access to each patient's specimen, the concept of rules-based testing or the application of algorithms can be effectively operationalized. In addition, those rules or algorithms can be driven from short-term and long-term outcomes-based approaches.

SPECIMEN TRANSPORTATION

The transportation of specimens throughout the laboratory is highly dependent upon the specimens that are procured and submitted (13–16). Specimens that are delivered to the laboratory can be separated into two general categories: (a) those that are cylindrical or tubular and (b) those that come in regular sizes and shapes, such as blood culture bottles, sputum containers, biopsies, glass slides from Pap smears, and so on (Fig. 7-7).

The specimens obtained in tubes are collected based upon the needs of the laboratory (driven by instruments) and the condition of the patient. Evacuated blood collection containers come in multiple sizes and shapes and contain a variety of different additives or no additives at all. In a hospital environment, the clinical laboratory cannot set a standard for the specimen collection containers or restrict the spectrum of specimen containers.

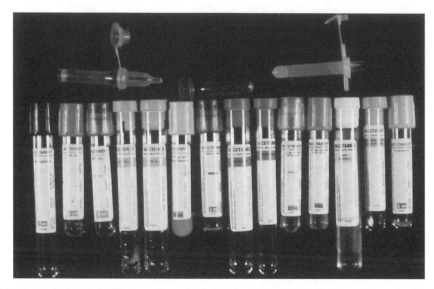

FIG. 7-7. A photograph of the spectrum and variety of containers that may be submitted to the laboratory.

This lack of standardization on one tube size requires that the clinical laboratory, especially in a hospital environment, be prepared to handle all sizes and shapes of evacuated blood collection containers. To deal with this issue, we developed a specimen transportation carrier that holds all the different sizes of tubular specimen containers currently in use, including pediatric specimen collection containers and glass slides. In addition, the carrier's external structure is physically defined and the internal structure is flexible so that carriers may be adapted to different payloads.

AUTOMATION SYSTEMS ISSUES

One of the most significant issues to deal with is unique specimen identification and the information required to make clinical and routing decisions based upon the tube label. The current LIS technology that has proliferated for the last 16–20 years and that currently exists in most clinical laboratories relies on the use of an accession number, the specimen number on the tube (number on the bar code label) that provides the link to orders and patient results. This accession number usually represents an episode of care or a series of orders and is not a unique identifier in all cases. The paradigm of computer-integrated manufacturing, which we are following in the implementation of clinical laboratory automation, requires that each tube be labeled with a unique identifier, such as a part number. The cost of changing the LISs from an accession number to a specimen number is staggering. Estimated costs would be somewhere between $200 and $800 million.

To overcome this problem, we put a unique identifier on the carrier. Our approach results in a unique identifier for each specimen in the laboratory by linking the specimen and matrix to the carrier number. There are several other advantages to having a label on the carrier, including the ease of reading a bar code on a flat surface versus the difficulty of reading a bar code on a curved surface or arc, such as the side of a tube.

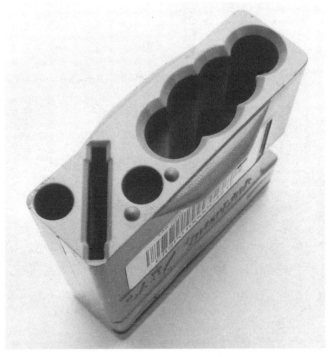

FIG. 7-8. A photograph of the LAB-InterLink, Inc. specimen carrier.

Another important issue is the ability of the specimen carrier to contain a fluid leak. Most current manufacturers of automation technology, as well as most of the rack-based or quadrant-based clinical laboratory instruments, use a system that allows fluid to leak through the carrier or rack. When a human operator is present, this is not as significant as when the process is automated. The human operator will notice a leak or a fluid spill and contain the biohazard. An automated system, however, does not have the means for detecting a fluid leak. In the absence of human intervention, a tube or specimen that is leaking on a transportation system will cause a significant amount of aerosolization. This could contaminate the entire laboratory, if no intervention occurs. To eliminate this problem, we built a carrier that has a capacity of slightly more than 20 ml to contain any fluid leaks (Fig. 7-8). The largest evacuated blood collection container used for specimens other than blood culture materials is a 15-ml tube. The entire volume of a specimen could be contained within the specimen carrier.

TRANSPORTATION HARDWARE

Transportation systems are another important consideration with respect to implementation of automation. A specimen transportation system is simply an enabler for the software that oversees the automation process. Many of the people who are currently investigating laboratory automation, either from a developmental standpoint or with respect to a purchase, focus on the hardware when, in fact, clinical laboratory automation is a software problem. This is not to say that the hardware is unimportant. We believe that it is and have engineered a 12-piece modular remove-and-replace system that can be configured to fit into any laboratory environment.

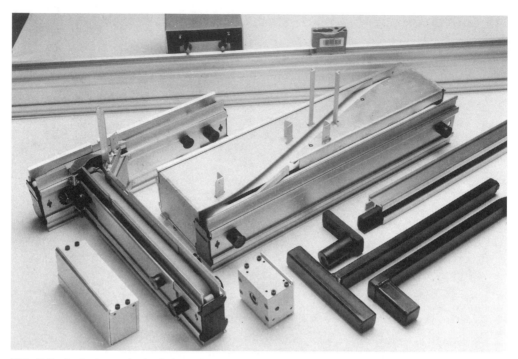

FIG. 7-9. A photograph depicting piece modular transportation system by LAB-InterLink, Inc.

The modular transportation system that we have created can be suspended from the ceiling, mounted on the wall, mounted as a belt line on the floor supports, or run underneath a subfloor, such as the floor that may be found in a computer room. The flexibility of the system allows the transportation system to conform to the shape of the room, as opposed to spending a considerable amount renovating the physical plant (Fig. 7-9).

The specimen transportation system is simple and flexible enough that all the components can be replaced by medical technologists or other technicians within the laboratory without any additional assistance. The only piece, however, that requires two or more people to remove and replace is the elevator mechanism.

The transportation system hardware components are monitored from the LAS software. Any error in the operation of the track system is documented by the software and the operator is notified through a paging system.

UPFRONT SPECIMEN PROCESSING

The issue of upfront specimen processing is difficult to understand. From 1993 through 1995, several articles were printed in *CAP Today* recounting the benefits of upfront specimen processing, which was defined as centrifugation and potentially aliquoting, as well as sorting. Several manufacturers—including IDS of Japan (marketed by Coulter Corporation, Miami, Florida) and Automed (a subsidiary of MDS Laboratories, currently located in Vancouver, British Columbia)—developed automated processes. The main premise of the IDS system was that a single tube size would be used for each processing line. This is a fairly unrealistic situation given the flow of specimens through the front end or specimen-receiving/specimen-processing areas in hospital laboratories. A single tube size is possible in reference laboratories or cultural situations where the pathology laboratory director can designate the tube size to be used in an institution or organization.

The Automed solution was developed for MDS Laboratories, Canada's largest clinical laboratory operation. This system is composed of several modules that centrifuge, aliquot, and sort several types of specimens. Reference laboratories or commercial laboratories are significantly different from hospital clinical laboratories.

The primary issue in the hospital clinical laboratory is that we must take all comers. We have the ability to designate preferred tube sizes; however, of the 11 different tube sizes currently in production, four are most commonly used. Those tube sizes are 13 × 100, 16 × 100, 13 × 75, and 16 × 75.

It is doubtful that we will be able to consolidate specimen collection into fewer than these four frequently used tube sizes. It is therefore highly unlikely that a single tube size could be used in the hospital laboratory routine clinical practice that would be facilitated by the current automation technologies available for specimen processing. Thus specimen processing should be developed from the prospective of the needs of both the patient and the laboratory. What may be a reasonable solution from an engineering viewpoint may be impractical in health care delivery.

INSTRUMENT INTERFACES

One of the most significant issues in the automation of the clinical laboratory is control over the operation of the instrument. We have defined a concept called the *docking device*. The docking device consists of an electronic and mechanical interface with the instrument. The mechanical interface defines the movement of specimens onto, into, or through an instrument (Fig. 7-10). The original applications in our automation project fo-

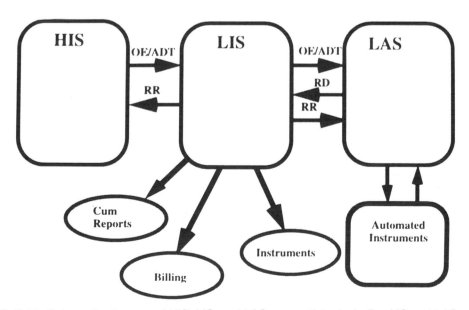

FIG. 7-10. Schematic diagram of HIS, LIS, and LAS connectivity, including LIS and LAS connectivity to instruments (ADT = admission, discharge, transfer; OE = order entry; RD = unverified results; RR = verified result reporting).

cused on the use of an articulated robotic arm to load and unload instruments. In 1991 we proposed the use of internal robotic devices by instrument manufacturers to load and unload their instrument in an effort to promote cost-effective health care. By using the internal automation technologies that exist in almost every clinical laboratory instrument currently marketed today, we could eliminate an articulated robotic arm and robot controller costing $30,000 to $60,000. Several instruments currently use drive-through specimen sampling, including the Johnson & Johnson VITROS 950 and 250 analyzers, the Chiron Centaur immunoassay analyzer, and the Technicon Dax series of chemistry analyzers. Many instrument manufacturers are currently working on automated specimen sampling interfaces analogous to the Johnson & Johnson VITROS series AT (automation technology) interface.

Instrument control is a much more difficult problem. The electronic component of the proposed docking device would allow for the current LIS download and upload of orders and results, as well as electronic control over the instrument. Our original concept was to parallel the approach currently used in computer-integrated manufacturing where there is control over the "machines" in the production line or on the factory floor. The control over these instruments is complex because of the nature of the instrument and the laboratory operation. Ideally, all the signals and/or messages that are sent to the screen and all the operations that could be performed through a screen or terminal should be possible using an electronic instrument interface. Johnson & Johnson has created this functionality for the interface to the VITROS series analyzers. Abbott Laboratories has worked on a version of software for the Axsym immunoassay instrument, and several other manufacturers are working toward this end. Adequate control of the instrument through some type of automation protocol is essential if clinical laboratory automation is to function.

THE "VALUE ADDED" OF THE TECHNOLOGIST

One of the most important lessons we have learned in clinical laboratory automation is that automation is not simple. Most of the early pioneers did not take into account the importance of the technologist in the production of quality laboratory results and information. They thought they could extract the technologist from the results production equation and simply provide a mechanical solution. It was clear to us several years ago that the process of producing results included the technologist and that we could therefore not extract the technologist from the equation without adding some type of "processor" to emulate the function of the technologist.

The technologist functions as a complex "CPU," processing inputs from both the instrument and the specimen against complex clinical rules and understanding of the technology. To make the LAS operate, we devised a software subsystem that takes inputs from the instrument, including status and errors, as well as inputs from the specimen, including state of the specimen and possible changes in the specimen to make decisions about the utility of the results. This process is only accurate up to a point, that being the utility of the programs and the adequacy of the information captured. When the limits of the functionality of the program are reached, the technologist is required to enter into results production even in an automated situation.

AUTOMATION SYSTEMS SOFTWARE

The software for clinical laboratory automation is the most important part of the process. The process control software to run an automated clinical laboratory functions as a "process" umbrella over the entire laboratory and should interface to the LIS. This umbrella of software will take into account results from different parts of the laboratory, including those portions of the laboratory that may not be automated in terms of specimen processing, specimen transportation, and results production. It is very clear that clinical laboratory results and their relationships are independent of the technologies that can be easily automated.

In our current LAS architecture, the automated instruments are interfaced directly into the LAS software. The LAS software is then interfaced into the LIS for the receipt of orders and admit discharge transfer (ADT) as well as verified results. Unverified results are transmitted from the LAS to the laboratory information system, where the LIS procedures for validation and release of results occur.

The LIS is used to interface to nonautomated instruments, to produce interim and cumulative reports, and to bill. An LIS is usually interfaced to a hospital information system (HIS) (Fig. 7-11).

As discussed earlier, the LAS, if designed correctly, will allow for implementation rules for the purpose of utilization management. Utilization management may occur at

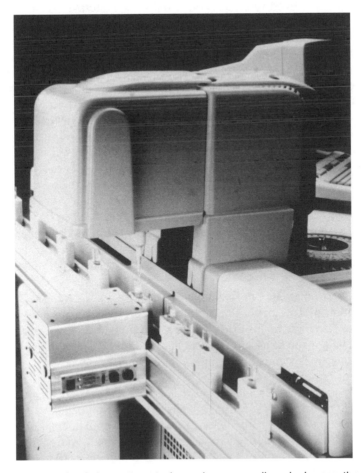

FIG. 7-11. A photograph of the automated specimen sampling device on the Johnson and Johnson Vitros 950AT Chemistry instrument.

the laboratory level or at the hospital level, with the laboratory being one subcomponent. The architecture of the database is important, if not critical, in the development of adequate utilization management schemes.

DECIDING WHICH TECHNOLOGY TO IMPLEMENT

Deciding which laboratory technologies to automate is difficult. Clinical laboratories in general have the same mission; however, they are not designed in the same way nor do they employ the same instruments.

Several categories can be automated to form the core laboratory, including chemistry, hematology, immunoassay, urinalysis, and coagulation. The automation of these areas of test results could account for 60% to 80% of the test results produced in the laboratory. By implementing a flexible automation technology that is information system driven, significant savings could be seen in the laboratory at several levels, including (a) reduction in FTE balanced against a 3–5-year amortization of your technology investment; (b) implementation of utilization management algorithms or rules-based protocol to optimize the sequence of testing or series of test results produced for a specific diagnosis or patient; and (c) delivery of clinical laboratory information that may be utilized in an integrated delivery system or for the production of outcomes data.

Utilization management, optimized outcomes, and information that links into an outcomes-based information strategy are far more valuable than simple return on investment for the automation purchase. It is clear that the current visionaries in outcomes optimization and outcomes-based information technology are seeking automation that is information system driven and that complements their information strategy.

The selection of a LAS must be determined by the needs of the laboratory on the health care delivery system or both. The selection of a software-based system such as the AutoLab or the LAB-InterLink solution will most likely be driven by the need to integrate laboratory information throughout the enterprise. The software-based systems allow for the implementation of real-time rules-based processing and support utilization management.

The selection of a hardware-based solution such as the Coulter/IDS or Hitachi/BMC solution will most likely be driven by high volumes of a limited number of tube sizes. The hardware-based systems most closely approximate the physical work of the laboratory technician. Payback models for the hardware-based systems have been gathered primarily in Japan.

The hurdles in clinical laboratory automation are not a surprise. The change induced by implementation of automation technology in the clinical laboratory is difficult for many to accept. Requests for justification data and guarantees by clients and potential clients are met with a spectrum of data. The hard data required to adequately justify the cost of a LAS have not been delivered, nor will they be for the next year to a year and a half. Several innovators and early adopters have selected technology based upon their understanding of the parallels in industry and computer-integrated manufacturing. Until 20–50 LASs are operating in a spectrum of laboratory environments we will not have sufficient data to document and justify the costs of purchase, implementation, and operation. In addition, the slower the industry is to adopt laboratory automation, the less likely the prices are to fall rapidly. To make a sound decision to purchase a LAS, you must decide whether you and your staff have the risk tolerance to implement a technology that is new to the laboratory.

FUTURE APPLICATIONS

One of the other important issues is the ability of the market or potential market to see cooperation between vendors of laboratory automation and instruments. It is very important for one or more of the instrument manufacturers to develop a solution for laboratory automation that could be seen as a "starter set." Johnson & Johnson Clinical Diagnostics has taken this leadership position by forming a three-way alliance with the leaders in clinical laboratory automation, LAB-InterLink (Omaha, Nebraska), Coulter Corporation (Kendall, Florida), and Johnson & Johnson Clinical Diagnostics (Rochester, New York) to produce a composite chemistry work cell. The chemistry work cell will include a Coulter IDS automation hardware and transportation system, including an input station, centrifuge, output station, and optional aliquoter. The hardware will support one to five VITROS instruments that have direct track sampling capability (the AT series). The hardware and instruments will be controlled by the LAB-InterLink automation software system that will interface the IDS/Coulter hardware components, the Johnson & Johnson Clinical Diagnostics VITROS instruments, and the LIS.

CONCLUSIONS

Clinical laboratory automation is a complex combination of information systems and hardware. The key to creating viable clinical LASs is a thorough understanding of the fundamentals of the clinical laboratory operation and the health care delivery system and applying the appropriate technologies to solve the problems.

Clinical LASs will continue to develop and mature. The technology will advance only if early adopters and risk takers enter the marketplace. Smaller, more affordable "starter sets" of automation technology, such as the Johnson & Johnson clinical chemistry work cell, should move the market forward. Potential buyers of clinical laboratory automation technology should understand the business and clinical needs, as well as the technology at hand. Innovative technology development usually does not occur in large companies. The small start-up companies have the ability to move new concepts and ideas forward and are usually agile. Concentrate on the technology, not the size or name of the company, and the right answer will prevail.

REFERENCES

1. Sasaki M: The belt line system—completely automatic clinical laboratory using a sample transportation system. *Jpn J Clin Pathol* 1984;32:119–126. In Japanese.
2. Sasaki M, Sonobe H, Koresawa S, Nishida M: An attempt at transporting laboratory samples. The establishment and further development of the belt line system. *Jpn J Clin Lab Autom* 1985;10:82–90. In Japanese.
3. Sasaki M: The robotic system of the clinical laboratory. *Jpn J Clin Pathol* 1987;35:1072–8. In Japanese.
4. Sasaki M: How to make and manage clinical laboratory systems using robotic facilities. In: Okuda K, eds. Proceeding IUPAC 3rd International Congress. *Automation and new technology in the clinical laboratory*. London: Blackwell Scientific Publications, 1988, pp. 97–101.
5. Sasaki M: A fully automated robotics laboratory in Kochi Medical School, Japan (Abstract). *Clin Chem* 1989;35:1052.
6. Ogura K, Sasaki M, Kataoka H, Nishida M: The innovative robot system for serological examination test and blood transfusion test: using Seiko RT-3000 robot. *Jpn J Clin Lab Autom* 1987;12:613–618. In Japanese.
7. Markin RS: The impact of transplantation on the clinical laboratory: experience at the University of Nebraska with bone marrow and liver transplantation. *Arch Path Lab Med* 1992;116(10):1004–1011.
8. Boyd JC, Felder RA, Margrey KS, et al: Use of a robotic arm for specimen handling in a remote, unmanned clinical chemistry laboratory. *Clin Chem* 1987;33:1560.
9. Felder RA, Boyd JC, Margrey K, et al: Robotic automation of the intensive care laboratory. In: Strimaitis JR, Hawk GL, eds.: *Advances in laboratory automation: robotics 4*. Hopkinton, MA: Zymark Corp., 1988, p. 533.
10. Felder R, Boyd J, Savory J: Robotics in the clinical laboratory. *Med Lab Prod* 1987;2:18.

11. Felder RA, Boyd JC, Savory J, et al: Robotics in the clinical laboratory. *Clin Lab Med* 1988;8:699–711.
12. Felder RA, Boyd JC, Margrey K, et al: Robotics in the medical laboratory. *Clin Chem* 1990;36(9):1534–1543.
13. Markin RS: Laboratory automation: an introduction to concepts and terminology. *AJCP, Pathol Patterns* 1992;98(4, Suppl 1):S3–S10.
14. Markin RS: Clinical laboratory automation: a paradigm shift. *Clin Lab Manage Rev* 1993;7(3):243–251.
15. Markin RS, Sasaki M: A laboratory automation platform: the next robotic step. *Med Lab Observ* 1992;24(10):24–29.
16. Markin RS: Implementing automation in a modern clinical laboratory. *Lab Info Manage* 1993;21(2,3):169–179.
17. Forrey AW, McDonald CJ, DeMoor G, et al: Logical observation identifier names and codes (LOINC) database: a public use set of codes and names for electronic reporting of clinical laboratory test results. *Clin Chem* 1996;42:81–90.

8

Point of Care Testing

David B. Nash, Annette M. Fernandez, Nancy R. Ryan, William P. Moffitt

Ongoing changes in the practice of medicine, spurred by significant shifts in reimbursement policy as well as rapid advances in technology, have produced an evolving trend in laboratory medicine. As fee-for-service payment methodology becomes a relic of the past, reducing the cost of services in a hospital environment becomes paramount (1). Under the variable, cost-plus system of reimbursement in place prior to the implementation of DRGs (diagnosis related groups) and TEFRA (Tax Equilization and Fiscal Responsibility Act) in 1983, the payer assumed all risk for the cost of operations of the provider network, the intensity of care, and the incidence of disease within a given population. The primary emphasis was on the availability of and access to care. The shift to the fixed episode-of-care model, or DRGs, put the provider at risk for the cost of operations and the intensity of care but left the payer at risk for the incidence of disease. In general, it provided avenues to shift the burden of cost overruns.

Today an increasing movement toward capitated, fixed payment per life further shifts the financial risk from the insurer or payer to the provider. The provider is at financial risk for the cost of operations, the intensity of care, and, for the first time, incidence of disease within a population. In formulating strategic and operational plans, this forces the providers, both hospitals and physicians, not only to consider the cost of operations and alternative operational structures, but also to keep their quality and longer-term implications of patient care, which contribute to the general health of the patient population. Clearly, the latter is a longer-term issue, and the most immediate impact on financial survival will come from the reassessment of operations. But this does cause providers to consider both the cost and the impact on clinical outcomes when adopting new technology.

The shift in health care today is from fixed costs to variable costs; from high capacity and overhead to leaner operations and patient-focused resources; and from technology for the sake of technology to technology supporting the restructuring of operations and improvements in patient care. In light of the growing need to improve efficiency, internal processes are being evaluated, restructured, and monitored. The shift of care to less expensive outpatient settings and the focus on minimizing fixed-cost operations have resulted in the reduction of staffed beds at most hospitals. The centralized hospital as the primary site of health care is being replaced by decentralized, multisite operations and ancillary services such as home care, outpatient clinics, and same-day surgery units.

The challenge for health care providers, especially those in the traditional hospital environment, is to adapt to this mandate for change without compromising the quality of patient care. Advances in technology have further complicated the cost/quality equation. Significant changes in both the provision of care and therapeutic protocols are evolving at an ever-increasing rate. Fiscal reality necessitates the evaluation of new technology on the basis of contribution to operational efficiency and to improvements in patient care.

Because outcomes analyses in diagnostic services such as the clinical laboratory can be complex, complicated by numerous extrinsic factors, the primary focus of assessment of new technology has become a contribution to the cost and efficiency of operations.

As a result of these new fiscal realities, hospital-based laboratories are reevaluating their operations. Although this is a long-term issue, it causes the provider to asses both the cost and the impact on clinical outcomes when adopting new technology. For financial survival, reassessment of such operations as clinical testing and resource utilization is very important. No longer viewed as an ancillary support service unit, the clinical laboratory has become a significant factor in the overall improvement of clinical operations and direct patient care. An episode of care is a complex event involving a variety of interdependent clinical resources and operational logistics. The flow and timely availability of information are critical components in the cost-and-quality equation.

This new financial paradigm of managed care, coupled with increased acuity of patient conditions, has led to a focus on such critical variables as turnaround time (TAT) of laboratory tests, along with cost-effectiveness (CE) of therapy as part of the strategy to improve medical care of critically ill patients (2). Regulatory requirements demand that more attention be given to overall quality issues of patient care. In the laboratory, these pressures translate into requests to improve service for patients in emergency, hemodialysis, trauma units, and various other departments that rely on their testing results. These requests come out of a need to make improvements in the efficiency of clinical staff and reductions in clinical decision cycle time. It has been shown that a primary cause of delay in the review of STAT test results is the involvement of clinical staff in other duties subsequent to ordering analyses (3). Presumably, the unavailability of immediate results or unpredictability of the timing of test results causes the clinician to move on to other duties until results are available. Various operational clinical mechanisms have been developed to shorten TAT and meet those needs—for example, pneumatic tube systems to improve specimen transport to centralized laboratories, establishment of specialized STAT laboratories, and use of point of care testing (POCT) devices (4).

Point of care testing devices have emerged as an operational alternative to more traditional approaches to improvements in service such as STAT laboratories, which compromise the need for cost reduction. The reduction of costs in an operational environment that depends upon volume to absorb high overhead, coupled with the cost of specialized labor, is in direct conflict with the decentralization of traditional operating processes or the dedication of resources to be at-the-ready in centralized settings. This chapter aims to define POCT, examine its components of cost analysis, and determine the pros and cons of its use in different areas. Several studies highlighting these issues with regard to POCT utilization have been addressed. Different areas, such as emergency, bedside glucose testing, intensive-care unit (ICU) testing, and hemodialysis have been evaluated. By presenting the protocols and methodologies of different investigators and users of POCT devices we have compared the relative cost and service level of different POCT process implementations.

Special emphasis has been placed on cost in POCT because it has been a subject of great controversy. Literature has been interspersed with conflicting justification of both the presence and lack of benefits associated with POCT in a hospital. The improvements in clinical outcomes and resource utilization demonstrated in the literature have addressed only some of the critical variables necessary to measure valid outcomes. At the present time, when it is difficult to ascertain all necessary variables to do a complete, unbiased study of the cost-effectiveness of POCT, these studies provide some overview of the pros and cons associated with incorporating clinical testing into routine testing at a patient's bedside.

Critics hold that the cost of implementing POCT is supplemental to existing laboratory operations. This increases cost and therefore must be evaluated economically in light of improvements in patient outcomes. Proponents counter that this perspective ignores the implicit value in the point of care model through the redesign of process flows and that labor efficiencies, both internal and external to existing laboratory operations, should neither be discounted nor be considered unattainable. Indeed, improved efficiency of human resources is one objective of the point of care model. Moreover, this redesign of process flow can improve the efficiency of clinical staff by eliminating delay in clinical decision making and improving patient care through a reduction in decision cycle time. Thus, in principle, the savings in the cost of care could be even greater than the operational savings in cost per test, because clinical costs are greater than laboratory expenses. This is the crux of the debate on the value of POCT in a time of intense financial pressure.

HISTORY OF THE ORIGIN OF POCT

Prior to the 1820s, clinical testing was not a systematic science. It began with routine testing of urine samples. This was supplemented in the early 1900s by the introduction of electrodes for measurement of biopotentials. Discovery of photometers resulted in quantification, which increased credibility of testing. Automated assembly-line processes began to appear in the 1950s with the implementation of standard laboratory protocols and procedures. This resulted in greater capacity and increased accuracy of the analysis. In spite of all these advances, data acquisition was very slow because the most technological advances focused only on the analytical test process.

The need to decrease pre- and postanalytical delays, especially in areas of critical care, resulted in the introduction of satellite laboratories in the hospital environment. Advances in microprocessor technology and microfabrication of biochemical devices using semiconductor chip manufacturing technology have resulted in instruments that enable incorporation of blood analysis into routine patient care, in a manner that is minimally intrusive to the patient care work flow. This led to the introduction of POCT in the health industry with the prime objective of redesigning the entire testing process and improving efficiency. One could argue that any test that allows a physician to complete the disposition of a patient during a single visit is significant, because it optimizes patient care, reduces demands on the physician's time, and potentially generates a benefit by decreasing length of stay in more costly acute-care environments.

DEFINITION

POCT has been defined as "any laboratory test performed outside the central hospital laboratory facilities" (2). This definition may become obsolete as the boundaries between operating structures grow less finite. In other words, one individual's point of care may be another's central laboratory. Regardless of physical locale or proximity to other testing locations and facilities, the point of care is at the patient's side. Therefore a more universally applicable definition would be "testing performed at the patient's side." As a test, one could ask whether a sample is removed from the patient's immediate locale for processing. The site is usually close to the patient (at the point of care), such as the bedside, the physician's office, ambulance, geriatric center, operating room, or wherever medical care may be necessary. The flow and timely availability of information are critical in the cost and quality equation. Within the scope of this definition concept of POCT, the physician, nurse, or other health care professional attending the patient can order a laboratory test, obtain the specimen, and perform the analysis, having a tremendous impact on patient outcomes.

Culturally, POCT is a shift from a highly specialized department-focused labor force to a multidisciplinary patient-care-focused staff. Operationally, it is the reorganization of remote (from the patient) laboratory-based analysis into the duties of health care professionals at the patient's bedside. From a laboratory worker's perspective, it relies on decentralization of certain laboratory functions, a shift from the performance of tests to the management of information, and the functional support of a decentralized testing network.

Whatever the perspective, it is a paradigm shift based upon technology that enables the integration of blood analyses into the routine of patient care. The end result of this diagnosis can facilitate medical decisions that guide emergency interventions despite little or no knowledge of the patient's medical history (5). Theoretically, this key goal is achieved by minimization of therapeutic cycle time, which optimizes diagnostic–therapeutic processes. The end result of this diagnosis can facilitate medical decisions that guide emergency interventions of patients despite little or no knowledge of their medical history (4).

In an ideal experimental environment, if test results are available to the clinician immediately at the POCT, decision cycle time can be reduced and that can translate into reduced cost of treatment. Thus, in principle, the savings in the cost of care could be even greater than the operational savings in cost per test since clinical costs are greater than laboratory expenses. This is the crux of the debate on POCT's usefulness in times of limited financial resources.

THE REGULATORY ENVIRONMENT

At the federal level, performance of POCT is regulated by Clinical Laboratory Improvement Amendments of 1988 (CLIA 88) (6). Various regulations may also be applicable at the state level. Additional standards, particularly for tests categorized as waived by CLIA 88, are set by the Joint Commission for Accreditation of Healthcare Organizations (JCAHO) and the Laboratory Accreditation Program of the College of American Pathologists (LAP-CAP). Personnel performing the test should have appropriate credentials and be effectively trained in sample acquisition and test performances. The testing so far is of moderate complexity, so that it could be performed with adequate training and availability of a qualified supervisor.

Appropriate quality control, external proficiency testing, and instrument maintenance must be performed and documented (7). The National Committee for Clinical Laboratory Standards (NCCLS), a subcommittee for POCT, drafted a guideline to establish testing uniformity. It addresses specific organizational approaches, cost issues, and quality control (8). Of note, many of the regulations regarding POCT are changing as technology advances and the clinical and laboratory communities continue to gain experience with this approach to patient care. The efficacy of POCT thus is reliable only if the testing guidelines are maintained.

POCT: ADVANTAGES AND DISADVANTAGES

Kost and colleagues provide an overview of the different POCT devices currently available, along with details of usage (9). They include blood glucose monitors, whole-blood analyzers, thrombosis/hemostatis tests, and nanofabricators. In the last 5 years of

POCT, demand for glucose monitoring has increased rapidly. Recent surveys showed an increase from approximately 50% (10,11) to as high as 75% in near-patient testing and 83% in the case of hand-held testing (12), with 87% of U.S. hospitals implementing POCT programs (13). A recent survey indicated that 79% of these hospitals implemented POCT with a view to improving patient care (12).

POCT devices perform many of the same tests done in the central laboratory. One advantage of using POCT is faster therapeutic intervention, with fewer steps in a hospital unit and in the lab test pathway. For example, Becker and colleagues demonstrated that in patients undergoing anticoagulation therapy, the availability of POCT coagulation results reduced the mean time to stabilization from 18.1 to 8.2 hours (14). At the same time, POCT requires only a small sample size of fluids and/or tissues. This results in increased convenience for the patients (15).

Implementation of this new technology within the framework of a centralized laboratory poses a major disadvantage if the test results need verification by the central laboratory. Duplication of tests often results in increased resource utilization that is detrimental to the health care organization. An accurate evaluation of the premise that POCT provides effective medical care because of decreased TAT must compare the operation of a POCT with a central laboratory. When assessing the financial impact of POCT, it is necessary to look at the entire cost of patient care, not just the cost of patient testing. Also, when assessing the economic impact of POCT, it is necessary to look at the entire cost of patient care, not just the cost of the tests.

ECONOMIC CONSIDERATIONS OF POCT

As with any new technology or prospective change in operations, there are many proponents of the benefits of this new technology. The cost of introducing POCT in any health environment must be accurately identified and assessed within the context of the required service level. Economic benefits are derived through an interdepartmental systems optimization rather than through the localized optimization of individual departments. Various analyses have been conducted that attempt to address this issue. But few studies start with the assumption that POCT is a supplement to existing laboratory operations, and not a tool for restructuring. For example, some analyses assume that laboratory costs are largely fixed. In other words, the testing workstation, attendant operators, and support costs would remain largely intact, and POCT costs would be additive, with the only offsetting cost being the decrease in the marginal costs associated with reagents and supplies, as a result of doing fewer tests in the lab. Thus such analyses compare fully loaded POCT costs with marginal laboratory costs. Also, in some analyses significant clinical department costs are attributed to POCT, whereas these same sources of cost are not captured and reported for the traditional laboratory process costs. Because cost is one of the primary issues determining the inclusion or exclusion of POCT in a hospital, we have addressed the total costs of creating a product that includes fixed, variable, and step function costs as well as operationally related costs such as clinical staff.

Fixed Costs

Fixed costs for diagnostic testing POCT are composed of the cost of space and its attendant support costs such as utilities, the labor of supervisors and management of the program (management, office help, laboratory technicians), equipment (purchased or rented), certain components of the quality system, supplies (medical/surgical and office), and department, inclusive of education and in-service training. Education of a large number of operators for appropriate handling of these POCT devices affects the cost, depending upon frequency of usage. These costs ensure the availability of the test irrespective of usage. Hence a low volume results in higher cost per test and vice versa. Because POCT devices have lower equipment and maintenance costs compared with traditional larger central laboratory equipment, they are more cost-effective from a fixed-cost perspective. When a large volume of tests are performed, total cost increases proportionally and cost per unit remains constant.

Variable Costs

Variable costs are associated directly with a specific test and are incurred solely as a result of performing the test. As a result, they are unit volume dependent. All these can be assigned specifically to the end product (16). These costs include the disposable supplies, consumable reagents, and chemicals used in each test procedure. The cost of labor to perform the test may also be applied as a variable cost if the labor component varies directly with unit volume. As will be demonstrated later, in traditional laboratory process flow, labor is more appropriately categorized as a step function cost. The labor to perform the test in the POCT model varies directly with unit volume and therefore can be considered a variable cost.

Step Function Costs

Step function costs vary with volume, but not on an incremental basis. Rather, this terminology is used to define those costs that vary with large increments of volume. Depending upon the ratio of the magnitude of volume in such an increment to the total volume of a given operation, these costs can appear to be fixed. An example of this is the cost of labor in a traditional laboratory setting, whether it is a central laboratory or a satellite STAT facility. The labor cost of the first technician required to run a given analyzer appears to be a fixed cost until a given level of volume is reached, thus requiring the addition of a second technician. Because the first technician is required to perform any tests, this initial component of labor may be considered fixed, with the cost of each additional technician more appropriately fitting the definition of a step function cost. Step function costs associated with diagnostic testing are the labor directly applied to the testing process, and the cost of certain components of the quality system.

Associated Hidden Costs

Analysis of other costs associated with the testing process depends upon several factors, not all of which are tangible or consistent for a given situation. It involves potential cost savings generated by affecting physician practice patterns, patient morbidity/mortality, surrounding environmental factors conducive or nonconducive to rapid TAT, presence or lack of effective communication in the hierarchy, and so on. Although less work has been done to document and quantify these costs, arguably these are the more significant costs because they are a by-product of the service level and are more directly associated with patient care.

The economic proposition of POCT is that these associated costs are reduced through improvements in service levels (TAT) while simultaneously reducing the cost of the testing process through the elimination of certain fixed and step function costs. Because most POCT systems involve variable costs that are greater than traditional testing processes, analysis of the total process is important.

Either a defect-rate-inclusive approach or a cost-centered approach can be used to determine costs of all testing processes, including POCT. The defect-rate-inclusive approach is based on total cost management and ascertains the preventive, appraisal, internal-failure, and external-failure costs associated with the system. Preventive costs are those associated with various mechanisms used to protect against process errors. These errors are personnel training, quality control testing, continuing education, and preventive maintenance. Appraisal costs are those incurred in ascertaining the degree to which a system meets its service requirements. Among them are proficiency testing, inspections and accreditation, and internal quality assurance audits.

Poor performance can result in specimen re-collection, repeat tests, confirmation by a second methodology, and results that are no longer relevant because of a lack of timely reporting. All these attribute to internal-failure costs. Poor performance outside the testing cycle incurred by the receiver of test results contributes to external-failure costs. All inappropriate clinical decisions based on excessive duplicate testing, STAT abuse, inaccurate, or untimely results are included in this category. The cost per unit of a POCT device is variable, depending on the device and the contractual agreements made. In an outpatient setting there is generation of revenue to offset the cost of utilization. However, in an inpatient setting, revenue must be reallocated from the hospital for the addition of any technology. Strict adherence to guidelines and suggested protocols can help in streamlining these costs.

In the business world, where total cost management is the norm for evaluating economic viability of any program, defect-rate-inclusive cost analysis is a standard tool. However, with POCT the benefits are not easy to quantify. The variables that need to be addressed are far too interrelated and complicated. As a result, this type of approach does not lend itself to a clinical setting and is sparingly adopted by hospitals. A cost-centered approach takes into account different fixed, step function, and variable costs. The problem lies in the evaluation of cost and benefits wherein the principal investigator decides on whether a true cost analysis should account for every single minute of labor time associated with POCT, or if it should also capture "free," structurally idle time.

As a result, one observes macroeconomic cost-centered analysis (total laboratory costs divided by test volume), wherein significant savings were observed when seven satellite laboratories were consolidated into one main STAT lab and two satellite laboratories (17). This further demonstrates the relatively high preponderance of fixed costs associated with traditional laboratory processes. As medical systems reorganize, some flexibility in certain of the settings remains that precludes application of a microeconomic analysis that accounts for every second of labor consumed.

In an era of decreasing reimbursements, where every laboratory and critical-care unit must evaluate cost and patient benefits to justify laboratory expense, one must also consider the outcomes for individual settings. From the outcomes point of view, some investigators have speculated that POCT produces an overall decrease in cost to the health organization similar to decreased length of stay. A true comparison of the cost-effectiveness of centralized laboratories versus POCT requires consideration of all aspects of care delivery, including staff, equipment, and supplies (4). Just as external-failure costs are affected by interrelated variables, outcome studies are even further compounded by the absence of a discrete link between test and patient outcome.

IMPACT OF POCT ON PATIENT CARE UNITS

Emergency

An emergency department is one of the areas in any health care system wherein faster laboratory results might be conducive to rapid clinical decisions and decreased length of stay (LOS), thus resulting in beneficial patient outcomes. Projections have been made regarding cost savings that can be generated by shorter TAT, LOS, and minimal labor, along with improved patient satisfaction. To understand the effect that technology has on quick patient recovery and the economics of care, outcome studies to assess the value of POCT throughout the continuum of patient care should be performed.

According to a study by Hutsko and co-workers, the impact of POCT on patient care and nursing in the Emergency Department highlights the fact that faster TAT ensured quicker diagnosis and treatment (18). The POCT analyzer used determined a patient's sodium (Na), potassium (K), chloride (Cl), glucose, blood urea nitrogen, and hematocrit value within 90 seconds. Physicians had quick results, and nurses spent less time waiting for laboratory results of critically ill patients and more time caring for those patients. Their cost analysis identified a premium when adopting POC rather than central facilities. However, POCT is used only 5% to 10% of the time. The authors have addressed the issue of "broader impact of improved patient and clinical staff management as a result of faster test results." However, this aspect has yet to be studied in full detail.

In a prospective study by Parvin and colleagues, the impact of POCT on patients LOS in a large emergency department was investigated (19). The hand-held POC device measured Na, K, Cl, glucose, and blood urea nitrogen during a 5-week period. Six other tests—pH, PCO_2, PO_2, calcium, hematocrit, and bicarbonate—though available on the same analyzer were not included in this study. LOS distribution during this experimental period (2,067 patients) was compared with that of a control setting (2,918 patients) for the same time frame prior to the institution of POCT and for 3 weeks after its use.

Median LOS, defined as the duration between triage (initial patient interview) and discharge or admission to the hospital, was 209 minutes for the experimental versus 201 minutes for the combined control periods. Stratification of patients based on present condition (e.g., chest pain, trauma, etc.), discharge/admit status, or presence/absence of other central laboratory tests did not reveal a decrease in the patient's LOS for any subgroup during the experimental period.

LOS data in this study agree with Saxena and co-workers (3), who evaluated the STAT orders to test serum electrolytes, glucose, blood urea nitrogen, creatinine, amylase and lipase levels, prothrombin time, and complete blood count (CBC). It was a two-phase study initially assessing baseline TAT, followed by a reassessment after implementation of the new laboratory information system and addressing unforeseen problems.

In the first phase the TAT for chemistry was 61 minutes from the time the specimens arrived in the laboratory and 70 minutes for CBCs from the time of accession. The longest component of TAT was delayed by physician review of the results (45 minutes). The second phase of the study found that the median within-laboratory TAT had improved to 36 minutes for chemical and 55 minutes for hematological tests. Other perceived components of TAT delay included preanalytic factors outside the control of the laboratory (e.g., blood sample collection and sending it to the laboratory, postanalytic delays in physician acknowledgment of the results).

The continuous quality improvement study resulted in a 41% reduction in median TAT for STAT chemical tests, measured from arrival in the laboratory. The analytic phase of overall TAT was reduced by 22% for STAT CBC requests and by 30% for chemical and other tests. The conclusion was that a dedicated STAT lab in the Emergency Department would not substantially improve TAT for the commonly ordered tests included in this study. This is in parallel to POCT, where the laboratory is physically in the Emergency Department.

These results differ from the reports of Sands and colleagues (20) and Tsai and colleagues (21). The study by Tsai and colleagues encompassed 210 patients of which 102 (48.6%) were admitted to the hospital and 108 were discharged from the emergency room. The physician's decision to discharge or admit a patient was based on Chem-7 or CBC laboratory values in 59 (28.1%) of the cases and on other factors in the other 151 (71.9%) patients. As a result, the 151 patients were not considered in this study. For the population that was followed, the impact of rapid TAT initiated an earlier intervention in 38 patients, whereas no effect was observed for 15 patients. Of the remaining six cases, two were excluded from TAT analysis because of incomplete data and the effect was indeterminable in the remaining four patients.

The cost model incorporated direct costs of labor, supplies, and depreciation associated with POCT and central laboratory testing services. Direct costs for supplies and depreciation, including acquisition and maintenance costs, were applied over the useful life of the equipment, which was estimated at 8 years for central equipment. Similar estimates were also performed for POCT equipment. Labor costs varied, depending on whether a nurse or a technician was drawing the blood and performing the test. Depreciation costs were based on acquisition and maintenance costs.

The cost estimated a low-end POC test volume of 14,160 (20%) and a high-end volume of 35,396 (50%), based upon the emergency census of 8,849 patients. Although the cost per test for low-volume POC tests performed by nurses or emergency technicians was $16.67 and $14.98, the cost for high volume was $16.15 and $14.37, respectively. The POCT turnaround time was a mean 7.4 times faster than the central laboratory (8 minutes compared with 59 minutes). After a therapeutic course was decided for the patient, physicians reported that POC testing resulted in earlier therapeutic action for 19% of the patients (40 out of 210 patients). Although their cost model did not calculate potential economic gains in the increased capacity for the Emergency Department patient, or admissions due to rapid TAT and increased throughput volume, it illustrated the savings to be realized in providing POCT services.

In many hospitals, blood gas analysis takes more than 30 minutes to complete, whereas electrolyte measurements can take between 15 minutes to a few hours. POCT allows for the direct measurement of critical analytes in whole blood and results in a TAT of 2 minutes or less (22). A study by Fleisher and colleagues suggests that in a tertiary-care medical center, a dedicated centralized laboratory equipped with a rapid-transport specimen system provides better comprehensive laboratory service than does a POC facility (23,24). The parameters that were considered during this analysis included TAT analysis for whole blood and measurement of serum analytes during a representative time period.

However, an analysis by Spoor suggests that costs are reduced by decreasing the number of lab test errors that have to be rerun and by the instantaneous availability of results (25). In POCT, both common variations (i.e., the standard deviation of waiting for results and uncommon variation due to excessive waiting because of sample mix-up) are low. As a rule, physicians are happier because of the faster results that enable prompt diagnosis and corrective actions, ultimately permitting them to treat a patient much more effectively. Faster TAT avoids a long wait in the Emergency Department caused by delayed diagnostic tests, thus contributing to greater patient satisfaction.

Cost Analysis of POCT by Component Analysis

I-STAT Corporation carried out a study to identify and quantitatively account for the components of primary service, TAT, and the full system cost of providing STAT tests from a variety of blood testing process models (26). This study was conducted in five hospitals to understand and develop effective automated cost planning tools for analysis of service level, along with associated costs of different cross-department blood-testing processes. The size of the hospitals ranged from 279 to 1,000 licensed and staffed beds. Three of these hospitals provided some or all of STAT blood analysis through staffed satellite laboratories in the critical-care unit. One of the hospitals used only a centralized STAT laboratory operating within and sharing the resources of the central laboratory. The remaining hospital used a combination of the central laboratory for some STAT tests and unstaffed satellite laboratories.

The sample group was unbiased and represented a variety of traditional approaches to STAT testing. These included dedicated STAT laboratories (as a part of the central laboratory) attended by personnel (with and without pneumatic tube delivery systems), departmental laboratories monitored and used by nurses and respiratory therapists, and centralized STAT facilities incorporated into the main laboratory, utilizing pneumatic tubes for specimen transport. The entire process for STAT and routine blood analysis was observed and documented on each operating shift and for all departments utilizing these services. Documentation for materials utilized and the costs incurred were meticulously recorded. The expenditure for supplies and disposables, maintenance costs, equipment depreciation, and labor costs were collected. Testing volumes were recorded for each entity. Different costs were computed, including total costs and cost per blood analysis. These were identified as fixed, step function in nature or variable directly related to volume.

The different tests included in this study consisted of Na, K, ionized calcium, glucose, hematocrit, pH, PCO_2, PO_2, and various specifically calculated parameters. External neutral auditors (not provided by the company) were assigned to make unbiased observations of all the preceding costs and processes. In addition to information on what materials were used and tasks performed, data were collected regarding the type of test ordered and the time allocated to perform each step of the testing process. In total, auditors spent more than 1,700 hours observing and recording approximately 1,000 patient blood analysis testing events within critical care units in the STAT and central laboratories. Direct labor costs were calculated for personnel who gave all or some of their time to the testing process. Interference that hindered the process flow (e.g., mechanical failure of pneumatic tube systems, clerical errors, and inadequate supplies) was recorded. Yearly expenses of fixed costs were collected, as were laboratory and patient costs.

Results indicated that the cost of the testing process (exclusive of physical plant and allocated administrative and institutional costs), which provided STAT blood gas and electrolyte services at each of the five hospitals, ranged from $217,764 to $779,856. Annual STAT test volumes associated with these processes ranged from $27,535 to $70,282.

Of the traditional approaches to STAT testing, the staffed satellite STAT laboratory model achieved the fastest TAT but exhibited the highest cost per testing procedure. Average STAT TAT for this model was 29 minutes, with a range of 14–46 minutes. Of the three hospitals utilizing this model, one exhibited a slightly lower cost per panel without any significant difference in the TAT and was the most efficient of all models encountered in the study. The one hospital providing STAT blood analysis from the central laboratory demonstrated the lowest cost per test performed but also the longest TAT (46 minutes). This is consistent with the cost/volume relationship of traditional operations. In comparison to a POCT model, the traditional methods of providing STAT testing service demonstrated higher costs and longer TATs regardless of model. The POCT model resulted in lower testing process costs by approximately 25% and a reduction in TAT of 82% from an average of 28 minutes to 5 minutes. Figure 8-1 demonstrates the cost of performing tests in a traditional STAT lab, comparing costs to volume.

Statland and associates advocate the use of the CALC (calculating annual lab costs) technique to compare costs of identical testing services with alternative testing configurations (16). This process involves identifying site locations with equipment configurations, tests offered, and number of samples expected to be processed. The cost of establishing and operating the entire testing service is recorded and annual testing cost is calculated. Although this methodology allows for the identification of direct and indirect costs, it does not evaluate nonintangible issues (e.g., the estimation of cost incurred due to the inability of a nurse to find a physician to transmit patient results in critical care) that heretofore have not been quantified in monetary terms.

Cost Analysis in a Community Hospital

The cost of POCT for glucose and electrolyte/glucose/blood urea nitrogen panel using the portable i-STAT analyzer by nurses was compared with that of performing the same analyses in a central laboratory (27). Cost calculations included labor, quality control, reagents, and indirect costs for administration, power, heat, housekeeping, and so on. Contributions of the pneumatic tube delivery system and the laboratory computer system were also factored into the calculations. The conclusion of this study was that in the case of already existing central laboratory capabilities, POCT exceeds central costs by a factor of from 1.1 to 4.6. According to their results, POCT proves to be a more expensive way of delivering rapid laboratory services (27).

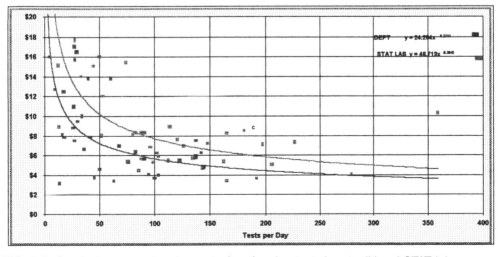

FIG. 8-1. Graph demonstrating the cost of performing tests in a traditional STAT lab comparing cost to volume. Dept: $y = 24.294x^{0.2711}$. Stat Lab: $y = 48.719x^{-0.3845}$.

POCT in a Pediatric Hospital

Diseases that affect children progress faster than they do in adults. In a retrospective analysis, Lynch reported that all participating hospitals performed POCT (28). Although 11% of the 46 institutions reported a decrease in their POCT, 61% reported an increase, and more than 74% of the respondents expected an increase within 3 years. The author used a total of 14 Likert Scale statements to determine the opinions of laboratory managers and directors about various POCT issues. Fifty-three percent of respondents viewed the cost of POCT as higher than that of central laboratory testing, whereas 30% disagreed with that premise.

Fifty-nine percent reported that POCT did not result in STAT requests, and 22% stated that their requests were down. In contrast to the high percentage (65%) reporting successful bedside testing, only 39% of all hospitals stated that their POCT results were accurate and reliable; 39% were neutral, and 22% perceived their results as inaccurate and unreliable. Although small sample size is one of the favorable characteristics of POCT, 58% did not find it a key factor in the decision to use POCT in a pediatric setting. This study indicates that laboratory directors and/or managers who participated in this survey had not reached a comfort level with the quality of POCT results. A large number of hospitals perform bedside-activated clotting time tests in addition to the widely performed tests such as glucose and fecal occult blood. The overall consensus is that pediatricians, who spend more time at the patient's bedside, are more apt to perform POCT than some other physician groups.

POCT in ICU

Although bedside hemoglobin and/or glucose measurements have been used for many years, most ICUs do not have comprehensive POCT that encompasses blood gas and electrolyte measurement at the bedside. Castro and colleagues addressed the significance of POCT in such a critical environment (29). POCT can decrease laboratory analysis errors originating in the ICU such as inappropriate specimen phlebotomy, identification, packaging, handling by ICU, transport, and so on. Sensor drift is diminished because of calibration with every sample. Analytical artifacts due to hyperlipidemia and hyperproteinemia are eliminated as a result of whole-blood measurement. Cost of care in the ICU could be decreased by earlier diagnosis, rapid therapeutic assessment, shortened LOS, and more efficient use of ICU, laboratory, and transport personnel (29).

A study by Zaloga investigated the average time to wean an uncomplicated postoperative patient from a ventilator, along with other parameters such as average ICU and hospital stay as well as average hospital cost in a group of patients treated with a bedside oximeter and those monitored with blood gases in an ICU laboratory (30). It was observed that bedside monitoring decreases weaning time, ICU stay, total hospital stay, and hospital costs. Bedside blood glucose monitoring with dry chemistry reagent strips was found to provide an accurate assessment of blood glucose levels when performed by nurses. A decrease in the cost of monitoring blood glucose levels and hospital stay in diabetics was observed when bedside testing replaced laboratory testing (30).

LABORATORY AND BEDSIDE EVALUATION
Hemodialysis

Prior reports suggest that the use of POCT devices for assaying Na, K, Cl, urea, glucose, and hematocrit gives values that are similar (smaller standard deviation than central laboratory) to those of accepted central laboratory methods, and have comparable precision, even when determined by nonlaboratorians (31). Gault and co-workers stated that the preceding parameters, along with pH and ionized calcium, can be assayed acceptably in the dialyzate fluid used for hemodialysis (32). The mean differences between POC and central laboratory values were 0.2% for hematocrit and 3.1% for urea, and higher values for ionized calcium (4.3%) and glucose (11%) were observed.

Their preliminary data suggested that sodium, potassium, chloride, hematocrit, urea, and pH can be assayed acceptably in the dialysate fluid used for dialysis. Such POC analysis may have particular value for patients with kidney failure in the Emergency Department.

Thrombosis

Use of lysis-onset time (LOT) measurements with test cards containing thrombotic agents, such as thrombin or batroxobin, provides a global fibrinolytic test. Patients who should not be given streptokinase or antistreplase could be identified before therapy, as could patients requiring higher doses to overcome neutralizing antibodies. This type of rapid POC test is very useful in estimating resistance to streptokinase and other drugs (33).

POCT by Medics Prior to Hospitalization

Although prehospitalization assessment is crucial in sustaining the vital signs of a critical patient, not many studies are devoted to analyzing the effectiveness of POCT in such situations. Herr and colleagues studied a helicopter program for transporting critical patients to evaluate POCT (34). They reviewed the value of POCT in the field, which allowed the crew to intervene immediately and possibly deliver a more stable patient to the emergency room. A POCT analyzer was used on 81 patients transported by flight crew. The tests performed included Na, K, glucose, and hematocrit/hemoglobin concentrations. Comparison studies were performed on patient samples drawn and analyzed in the helicopter and subsequently analyzed in the hospital satellite lab and clinical chemistry laboratory.

No differences were observed in the performance of the POCT instruments versus those in the central laboratory. Discrepancies in the glucose results were associated with the time lag between collection and analysis in the helicopter, and subsequent analysis in the laboratory, estimated to be 30–45 minutes. Fifteen (18.5%) of the patients were treated with transfusions, glucose, or insulin based on POCT testing results. Twenty patients (24.7%) were given a treatment other than intravenous fluids, such as normal saline or Ringer's solution. One patient with leukemia was administered fresh-frozen plasma and platelets based on the hemoglobin value (60 g/L).

These initial findings look promising for improving the care of patients in the future. Other potential applications include arterial blood gas analysis (under evaluation) in helicopters and fixed-wing aircraft, and other analytes such as magnesium and lactate. One can see the potential application for transporting neonates, because minimal blood volume is required for analysis. One can envision the application of such new technologies extending to the prehospital environment.

Glucose Monitoring

Diabetes mellitus is a disease on which $10 billion is spent each year. Most of that expense relates to hospital care for treatment of complications. Because blood glucose is a moving target, timeliness of blood glucose results is particularly relevant. However, given the relative imprecision of therapeutic efforts, accuracy and precision of the blood glucose assay are of limited importance compared with timeliness. Having a bedside test that ensures that a patient's blood glucose level is within 10% to 15% of the true value in 1–2 minutes is more valuable than learning the exact blood glucose level an hour or more after the fact (35). The clinician can respond rapidly to changes in the patient's blood glucose levels, resulting in optimum insulin regulation and shorter, less expensive hospitalization.

Nichols and colleagues conducted a two-phase laboratory and bedside evaluation of portable glucose meters (36). Precision, linearity, correlation to the laboratory method, interference from hematocrit, data management and operator preferences were the parameters assessed. None of the four meters was found to satisfy all the study's evaluation criteria. The evaluation in this report indicates that FDA approval and marketing statistics are insufficient to judge the performance of the meters in routine institutional use. The clinician must interpret near-patient glucose results with respect to the meter limitations.

Lee-Lewandrowski and colleagues studied the use and cost of bedside glucose testing in a large teaching hospital in a prospective study of 40 inpatient units and 10 outpatient units (37). The number of glucose monitors increased from 2 to 54 over a period of 2 years. In 1992, of the 67,596 tests performed at the bedside, 30.7% were glucose measurements. The average cost for all units using bedside testing was about 8.4% higher than the central laboratory. The cost varied, depending on the unit (median $5.52, range $3.08 to $48.16). Different components of the cost factor were labor (e.g., cost of the time required to perform a bedside test), consumables (e.g., cost of optimum use of supplies), and other costs (e.g., instruments, maintenance, indirect overhead rates, transport costs). Indirect costs such as space and utilities were not added. In the seven high-volume units, the costs per test were lower than the corresponding laboratory cost.

The conclusion was that bedside blood glucose testing was not more expensive than centralized testing, but inherent implementation on inefficient care units with low-volume utilization could substantially add to the cost. The high costs have been attributed to quality control, quality assurance, training, and documentation. Suggestions for accurate adoption and implementation of POCT are also addressed by the authors.

Troponin Evaluation

Antman and co-workers evaluated a rapid, qualitative bedside immunoassay for cardiospecific troponin T (cTn), using a hand-held device containing monoclonal antibodies (38). This assay is a qualitative assessment for a serum cardiac marker. They compared this assay with the clinical standard for diagnosis of myocardial infarction (MI) in a tertiary-care university medical center. A cohort of 100 patients was admitted for evaluation of chest pain. The outcomes measured were sensitivity and specificity of rapid cTn assay for MI, ratios of positive and negative rapid cTn assay result, and relative risk for serious cardiac events after admission.

Sensitivity of the cTn assay increased from 33% within 2 hours from the onset of chest pain to 86% after 8 hours. Specificity ranged from 86% to 100% in the same time interval. The odds of MI increased sixfold with a positive assay result within 2 hours of chest pain and decreased sixfold with a negative assay result after 8 hours. This finding is particularly important when evaluating a patient with a nondiagnostic electrocardiogram due to a previous Q-wave myocardial infarction, bundle branch block, preexcitation, or ventricular pacing. It endows the physician with a useful laboratory tool for bedside triage and prognostication of patients with chest pain syndromes and may have a significant impact on health care delivery in the emergency and coronary care units. Eisenbrey addressed the lack of cost data on cTn utilization (39).

No studies have been reported addressing cost issues and the technical expertise necessary to perform this assay. At the same time with the incidence of both false positives and false negatives, the probability of this test being repeated in the central laboratory is very high. In the present era of limited funds where one addresses cost-effectiveness and cost benefits, this argument is circumvented by proposing utilization of this procedure in specific patients who meet predetermined criteria. In the case of hospitals unable to support full-time CK-MB analysis, this rapid assay could be beneficial.

CQI and POCT for Home Care

Gogola and co-workers established continuous quality improvement (CQI) techniques for approximately 6 years and guided the development and subsequent alpha and beta testing of POCT for ambulatory patients (40). The primary measure of increased productivity chosen was the ratio of aggregate agency payroll hours to the number of home visits performed. This measure included labor hours of employees whose functions were beyond the scope of the system (e.g., checking various paper forms for internal consistency). However, the benefits of electronic charts clearly go beyond direct patient care labor hours by the nurses.

Over a 10-month period, productivity increased by 20%. On an annualized basis this translated into a potential increase of home care revenue of $876,000, using the same staffing level, and an 83% reduction in billing errors. Although not directly measured, the project team attributed the improvement in the quality of charting to POCT in the home rather than in the office, which usually occurs some time after the care was delivered.

POCT and Integration of Information

Current information technology allows data to be interfaced and integrated, and patient processes to be enhanced through tracking of clinical outcomes and reducing costs. Jacobs and co-workers address the issue of data entry into medical records in a POCT environment (41). Their idea that patient-centered integration is the key to successful health care information and that greater acceptance of POCT has merit needs to be part of the medical record.

CONCLUSION

Insufficient outcomes data exist on whether tests performed in the laboratory are cost-effective, rather than those performed at the point of care. Published and unpublished cost analyses show some consistent trends. Reagent costs per test for POCT are often higher than those for laboratory testing. But overhead and labor costs may be decreased, particularly if laboratory space or personnel (or both) can be decreased. Increased personnel effort is necessary for POCT management. The volume of testing can also influence the cost because of higher reagent expense per test and more frequent test failure with less experienced operators. Although less work has been done to document and quantify costs, arguably associated costs are the more significant because they are a by-product of the service level and are more directly associated with patient care. Because most POCT systems involve variable costs that are greater in comparison to traditional testing processes, it is important to reiterate that analysis of the total process is important.

The current trend in most hospitals is to subcontract the laboratory work to larger laboratories. Although this incurs less financial liability and indemnity to the hospital, it leaves it with minimal need for central testing. Faced with such a situation, one wonders about space utilization and reassignment of the central lab space to other uses, and the installation of POCT in its stead.

The continuing shift in health care is to decrease costs, create leaner operations, and focus resources. Many internal processes are being reevaluated, restructured, and monitored. The new paradigm of health care promotes less expensive outpatient settings with minimization of fixed-cost operations, and reduction of staffed beds for most hospitals. A centralized hospital as the venue for primary care is being replaced by decentralized, multisite operations and ancillary services such as home care, outpatient clinics, and same-day surgery visits (42).

The ability to minimize TAT with the use of POCT can result in quicker decisions regarding patient admission and discharge, as well as earlier and more appropriate diagnosis, fewer tests, and shortened LOS. These savings, however, are implied, not documented. As a rule, physicians are happier because the faster results enable prompt diagnosis and corrective actions. This ultimately allows them to treat a patient more effectively and contributes to greater patient satisfaction. If hospital laboratories are to survive and prosper in the future, they will need to identify and implement new financial methods that can teach and control their true costs, as well as evaluate different techniques to improve cost-effectiveness and quality of life for patients (43). They have to be in a position to ascertain the entire cost of an episode of health care to survive and thrive in the health care system of the next century.

REFERENCES

1. Jacobs E: Is point of care testing cost effective? *Clin Lab News* 1996; ....
2. Santrach PJ, Burritt MF: point of care testing. *Mayo Clin Proc* 1995;70:493–494.
3. Saxena S, Wong ET: Does the emergency department need a dedicated stat lab? *Am J Clin Pathol* 1993;100: 606–610.
4. Hunter L: POCT: costly or cost-effective? *Med Lab Obs* 1996;27(9S):2–3.
5. Kost GJ: Guidelines for point of care testing: improving patient outcomes. *Am J Clin Pharm* 1995;104:S111–S128.
6. Erhmeyer SS, Laessig RH: Regulatory requirements (CLIA 88, JCAHCO, CAP) for decentralized testing. *Am J Clin Pharm* 1995;104:S40–S49.
7. Belanger AC: point of care testing: the JCAHO perspective *Med Lab Obs* 1994;26(6S):46–49.
8. Goldsmith BM: New POCT guide establishes testing uniformity. *Med Lab Obs* 1995;27(8S):50–52.
9. Kost GJ, Hague C: The current and future status of critical care testing and patient monitoring. *Am J Clin Pathol* 1995;104(1S):S2–S17.
10. Jahn M: CLIA after year 1: no help to patients and a hindrance to labs. *Med Lab Obs* 1994;26:20–26.
11. *Blood gas monitoring: economic assessment and market strategies*. Washington, DC: The Lash Group, 1992.
12. McAllister E: *Point of care testing report*. Plymouth Meeting, PA: IMS America, Health Care Division, 1994.
13. Bickford GR: Decentralized testing in the 90s. A survey of United States hospitals. *Clin Lab Manage Rev* 1995;8:327–338.
14. Becker RC: Bedside coagulation monitoring in heparin titrated patients with active thromboembolic diseases: a coronary care unit experience. *Am Heart J* 1994;128:719–723.
15. Linz WJ, Gillum R: Assessing the productivity component of cost: the College of American Pathologists laboratory management index program for alternative site testing. *Med Lab Obs* 1996;27(9S):17–18.
16. Statland BE, Brys K: Evaluating STAT testing alternatives by calculating annual laboratory costs. *Chest* 1990;97(5S):198S–203S.
17. Jacobs E, Sarkozi L, Coleman N: A centralized critical care (stat) laboratory: the Mount Sinai experience. *Crit Care Rep* 1991;2:397–405.
18. Hutsko GM, Jones JB, Danielson L: Using point of care testing to speed patient care: one emergency department's experience. *J Emerg Surg* 1995;21:408–412.
19. Parvin CA, Lo SF, Deuser SM, Weaver LG, Lewis LM, Scott MG: Impact of point of care testing on patient's length of stay in a large emergency department. *Clin Chem* 1996;42:711–717.
20. Sands VM, Auerbach PS, Birnbaum J, Green M: Evaluation of a portable clinical blood analyzer in the emergency department. *Acad Emerg Med* 1995;2:172–178.

21. Tsai WW, Nash DB, Seamonds B, Weir GJ: point of care versus central laboratory testing: an economic analysis in an academic medical center. *Clin Ther* 1994;16:898–910.
22. Jacobs E, Vadasaia E, Sarakozi L, Colman N: Analytical evaluation of i-stat portable clinical analyzer and use by nonlaboratory health care professionals. *Clin Chem* 1993;39:1069–1074.
23. Fleisher M: point of care testing: does it really improve patient care. *Clin Biochem* 1993;26:6–8.
24. Fleisher M, Schwartz MK: Automated approaches to rapid-response testing. *Am J Clin Pathol* 1995;104(S1): S18–S25.
25. Spoor PI: Traditional lab testing vs. point of care testing: comparing the costs. *MLO* 1996;27(Suppl 9):4–6.
26. Manuscript in preparation.
27. Nosanchuk JS, Keefner RT: Cost analysis of point of care laboratory testing in a community hospital. *Am J Clin Pathol* 1995;103:240–243.
28. Lynch SP: point of care testing in a pediatric hospital. *Med Lab Obs* 1995; 36–41
29. Castro HJ, Oropello JM, Halpern N: point of care testing in the intensive care unit. *Am J Clin Pathol* 1995;104(1S):S95–S99.
30. Zaloga GP: Evaluation of bedside testing options for the critical care unit. *Chest* 1990;97(5S):185S–190S.
31. Bach RP, Pedersen DH, Wong YW, Pysher T: Suitability of i-STAT portable analyzer for blood gas testing by laboratory and non-laboratory personnel. *Clin Biochem* 1995;28:361.
32. Gault MH, Harding CE: Evaluation of i-STAT portable clinical analyzer in a haemodialysis unit. *Clin Biochem* 1996;29:117–124.
33. Oberhardt BJ: Thrombosis and hemostasis testing at the point of care. *Am J Clin Pathol* 1995;104,1S:S72–S78.
34. Herr DM, Newton NC, Santrach PJ, Hankins DG, Burritt MF: Airborne and rescue point of care testing. *Am J Clin Pathol* 1995;104,1S:S54–S58.
35. Watts NB: Bedside monitoring of blood glucose in hospitals. *Arch Pathol Lab Med*;117:1078–1079.
36. Nichols JH, Howard C, Loman K, Miller C, Nyberg D, Chan DW: Laboratory and bedside evaluation of portable glucose meters. *Am J Clin Pathol* 1995;103:244–251.
37. Lee-Lewandrowski E, Laposata M, Eschenbach K, et al: Utilization and cost analysis of bedside capillary glucose testing in a large teaching hospital: implications for managing point of care testing. *Am J Med* 1994;7:222–230.
38. Antman EM, Grudzien C, Sacks DB: Evaluation of a rapid bedside assay for detection of serum cardiac troponin T. *JAMA* 1995;273:1279–1282.
39. Eisenbrey AB, Artiss JD: Cardiac troponin T and point of care testing for myocardial infarction. *JAMA* 1995,274:1342–1343.
40. Gogola M: A joint hospital/vendor project brings CQI and point of care teachology to home care. *Comp Nurs* 1995;13:143–150.
41. Jacobs E, Laudin AG: The satellite laboratory and point of care testing. *Am J Clin Pathol* 1995:104(1S): S33–S39.
42. Battelle Medical Technology Assessment and Policy Research Program: The economic and clinical efficiency of point of care testing for critically ill patients. *Med Lab Obs* 1996;27(9S):13–16.
43. Spoor PI: Traditional lab testing vs. point of care lab testing: comparing the costs. *Med Lab Obs* 1996;27(9S): 4–6.

9

Integrated Delivery System, Informatics, and the Laboratory: Managing Patient Service and Clinical Quality in a Complex and Evolving Health Care Environment

C. Martin Harris

The practice of medicine in the age of the integrated delivery system is becoming more complex from an administrative and clinical practice point of view. Hospitals, physician groups, and other health care providers continue to merge into organized delivery units, all designed to deliver enhanced patient service and improved clinical quality in a more cost-effective manner. As these groups expand, integrated information services, which support timely clinical decision making as well as broad views of member populations, are becoming a requirement (1). Successful health care delivery organizations of the twenty-first century will devise information management programs, providing a view of the continuum of care from any point in the delivery system.

The practice of laboratory and pathology medicine will be particularly challenged by the shift toward more integrated care services. More often the laboratory medicine division will be asked to provide clinical laboratory results in direct conjunction with other services or to become part of a larger information service, designed to provide broader clinical context (2). These requests will require the division of laboratory medicine to develop expertise in areas formerly the purview of traditional hospital information systems or external benchmarking organizations. Tools of information technology such as interface engines, meta databases, rules-based engines, and data repositories will be as integral to the practice of laboratory medicine as any specimen analysis (3).

This chapter will identify business functions in the health care marketplace that will encourage change, describe common information system strategies of the integrated delivery system, and review major technology issues that need to be addressed by a laboratory medicine division to meet the information requirements of these new organizations.

INTEGRATED DELIVERY SYSTEM BUSINESS INCENTIVES

The past 10 years have seen enormous change in the health care industry. As the national cost for health care continues to increase as a percentage of GDP (gross domestic product), all parties responsible for payments have responded with demands or initiatives to control expenditures while maintaining or improving the current standard of American health care (4). Federal programs (Medicaid, Medicare), commercial payers, and private employers have pursued multiple managed-care strategies—such as full capitation, specialty care, and point-of-service plans—as the principal mechanism for controlling expenditures. The implementation of such reimbursement programs has driven many of the organizational changes that are occurring today within the health care industry. Cost management is not the only factor driving reorganization in health care: changing attitudes about service and clinical quality have also resulted in new health care delivery system designs.

The integrated delivery system has been the most common organizational response to the business forces identified previously. Defined as the integration of all components of the continuum of health care services—including physicians, hospitals, home health, and management services—the integrated delivery system model will dominate many major markets in the United States by the year 2000. This will result in considerably fewer provider organizations caring for regional patient populations (4). These larger organizations will have the task of providing patient access to health care from any geographic point in the region while providing high-quality service in a customer-friendly fashion. Meeting these goals will require the development of information-based services that support cost-effective decision making in a distributed health care delivery system.

In response to these economic and organizational changes, clinical laboratories must develop the ability to deliver both clinical and information services, which are tightly integrated with the clinical process, as well as information management strategies of the integrated delivery system. As clinical guidelines, protocols, and disease management programs become more common, clinical laboratories will need to become the providers of patient- and disease-specific clinical results, which support the provision of high-quality and cost-effective care.

OPERATIONAL CHALLENGES FOR THE CLINICAL LABORATORY IN THE INTEGRATED DELIVERY SYSTEM

Health care provider organizations are currently changing into organized delivery systems, as described in the preceding section of this chapter. This evolution and new business process will result in the delivery of high-quality, cost-effective care, creating a new set of operational challenges for the clinical laboratory. The laboratory must address short-term, clinical processing needs while developing the infrastructure to support longer-term initiatives. However, several issues stand out as fundamental requirements for successfully managing during this period of change. In particular, member patient identification, resource utilization/clinical protocol management, and disease management will be important processes, ultimately defining the care model of the twenty-first century.

Member/Patient Identification

Integrated delivery systems are struggling with developing a uniform patient identification system that can be used to establish a record system. The national experience with the implementation of such a system has created a diverse set of operational solutions. Two approaches include the assignment of a universal identifier at the initial point of contact and coordination of disparate identifiers in a back office operation (5). The operational solution chosen by an integrated delivery system establishes the identifier scheme, with which the clinical laboratory must comply.

As an example, one major health delivery system in the midwestern United States has chosen to invest $10 to $30 million to produce a universal patient identifier at the point of initial contact with their member/patient. This is different from most organizations, which establish a common identifier when the coordination of service delivery requires such a number. In the first scenario, the clinical laboratory is in a position to create a clinical record of all services provided for the member and to provide valuable additional monitoring capabilities (i.e., screening results based on age, sex, and diagnosis) for the clinical staff. Generally, the creation of an accurate historical record of services is still a challenge. Although the first strategy adds obvious benefits throughout an integrated delivery system, the disparate numbering approach is still the most common identification system used at this time, because of design, time for development, and cost issues. As previously mentioned, the financial expenditures for an initial point-of-contact system are estimated to be in the tens of millions of dollars and the time for development ranges from 2 to 5 years, depending on the complexity of the design.

Resource Utilization and Clinical Protocols

Eighty percent of all health care expenditures result from orders placed by physicians or their surrogates. Many systems have been devised to assist clinicians with decision making in an attempt to control or reduce expenses. These support tools are designed to ensure that the most cost-effective diagnostic and treatment strategies are chosen, without compromising clinical quality.

The most well-known resource utilization techniques include resource access control, standardized diagnostic and therapeutic formularies, and clinical profiling (6). Resource access controls and standardized formularies are centralized control systems designed to limit utilization. These systems are very effective in reducing the utilization of costly, technologically advanced care approaches (7). However, a significant percentage of unnecessary utilization results from excessive use of common diagnostic and therapeutic interventions. Clinical profiles seek to reduce unnecessary utilization by providing clinicians with diagnosis-specific, case-adjusted feedback on their individual practices, as compared with those of their colleagues treating the same illnesses (8,9). Profiles establish variances at the component level of diagnostic and treatment plans, and allow the clinician to ascertain where their practice differs from other practitioners. Most clinical laboratories currently support these initiatives, because requests for information from the laboratory are limited to patient- and time-specific data.

The clinical protocol presents new challenges in information delivery for the clinical laboratory. Clinical protocols are developed utilizing expert clinical knowledge derived from the medical staff, nursing department, and other allied health professionals, all working together to establish best clinical practices (10). These groups utilize external clinical benchmarks, practice guidelines, and medical literature to establish optimal management protocols for selected patients. As these protocols become more prevalent in acute-care medical practices, the request for information from the clinical laboratory will become far more complex than that described in the previous discussion of resource utilization and clinical profiles. In this scenario, the laboratory must provide situation-specific clinical results that support medical decision making against established protocols in real time. It is no longer adequate to produce batched results files for lab analysis or standard laboratory department results reporting by patient; results reports that are part of an overall clinical management summary are required. To accomplish this goal, laboratory medicine practitioners and information specialists must support the creation of targeted results strategies. For example, in many institutions, protocol management of the preoperative patient has resulted in improved service, cost, and clinical process outcome measures (8). The laboratory has been an integral part of this success story by providing selected results for patients prior to the surgical procedure, integrated with the preoperative clinical protocol, resulting in medical and anesthesia clearance of the patient requiring surgery. This integrated medical information report has significantly reduced surgical cancellations and operating room process delays.

Disease Management

Extending the concepts of clinical protocols to management of the member/patient is the basis of disease management programs. Although conceptually similar to the clinical protocol, a disease management program addresses large populations over a wide geographic area, utilizing disparate clinical resources (8). The operational challenges for the clinical laboratory include delivering context-specific information to the appropriate end user, who may no longer be the ordering clinician, or the delivery system in which the clinical service was provided. The laboratory will be expected to work with numerous business units to provide the required information in the proper context. Many sponsors of disease management programs are not provider organizations at all. Several pharmaceutical firms have developed this methodology as a mechanism for better understanding their products in the clinical setting. Working closely with provider organizations, the pharmaceutical industry is developing the information technology infrastructure to distinguish its product's performance in the clinical setting (11).

INFORMATION TECHNOLOGY REQUIREMENTS FOR THE INTEGRATED DELIVERY SYSTEM

Expertise in information technology is a growing requirement for the clinical laboratory. To support the initiatives described in the preceding discussion a technological knowledge base must be developed that includes interface engines, orders management, enterprise data repositories, and Intranet/Internet technologies. This section will briefly define the technology and describe issues of deployment.

Interface Engines

Interface engines are commercially available and used for several purposes, including computer-to-computer connectivity, transfer of data sets, reconfiguration of data, and clinical decision support.

A common use of interface engine technology is establishing connectivity between two computerized information systems to accomplish data transfer (3). Historically, interface functions were the province of the interface group of information system vendor organizations. These groups supplied all components of an interface from protocol to hardware platform. Interface engines have dramatically reduced the time required to establish technical communications between two systems. In conjunction with the establishment of standard information exchange protocols such as Health Level 7 (HL7) and others, interface engines have also reduced the time to implement operation of differing machine interfaces. The interface engine can also be used to manage issues related to format difference between application programs. The interface engine is capable of identifying blocks of text from standard reports and transposing the segments to achieve the desired format of the end user. This technique is frequently used to produce customized results for clinical protocol-based result reporting.

The interface engine can also be used to execute or obtain other applications. An example of this capability is the automated results-management system. Utilizing the capability of the interface engine to identify specific blocks of text, results can be pulled from a standard report and analyzed by application programs designed to identify critical values and ultimately page the ordering clinician.

Order Entry

Order entry technology was primarily developed to improve the efficiency of clinical department ordering and charge capture for billing. Over the past 10 years this has become the basis for the automation of resource utilization and clinical protocol programs. Order entry has resulted in improvements in both clinical service and outcomes. In one study conducted at a major medical center, the implementation of an order entry system on one-half of the general medicine services resulted in a reduced gross charge per case of approximately $800 (12). Other benefits included improved order accuracy and decreased service turnaround times. In another study an order entry system was demonstrated to improve the clinical process of care. Analysis of preoperative ordering and medication charting patterns revealed that prophylactic antibiotics were being given to patients too far in advance of the surgical procedure. When operational changes were made to ensure that antibiotic administration occurred within 1 hour of the procedure, postoperation infection rates were reduced by 50% (8).

Order entry technology is constantly improving, and recent surveys have shown that more than 50% of academic medical centers have plans for clinician-driven order entry within the next 5 years. With this change clinical laboratories will be required to support order entry technology, thus improving resource utilization and clinical care. An understanding of how order entry systems actually post orders, perform conflict checking, handle cancellations, and interact with external knowledge bases is required to effectively implement the laboratory aspect of a clinical protocol. Several articles in the *Annals of Medicine* have demonstrated the efficacy of using an algorithm for the initial dosing and chronic administration of heparin (13). The algorithm is based on age, weight, and prior measures of the coagulation system. To support the automated implementation of this important clinical guideline, the laboratory must provide context-specific coagulation results that support the management of the therapeutic protocol.

Enterprise Data Repositories

Another common technology strategy being deployed by large health care providers is the enterprise data repository, designed to capture data from a myriad of systems that exist inside of these organizations. Traditionally, computerized health care applications have been developed along functional lines such as registration/scheduling, patient accounting, general financials (general ledger, accounts payable, etc.), order entry/results reporting, radiology, laboratory, and so on. Each of these applications has an associated database, constructed to support rapid transaction processing and limited reporting of departmental management information. It is frequently difficult, if not impossible, to perform broader program analysis, requiring data from all or most of the systems outlined previously. The enterprise data repository has developed in response to the need to perform the collective analysis. Implementation of a repository establishes an institutional data dictionary to which all incoming data must be mapped. Finally, this technology supports advanced industry standard query products, such as sequential query language (SQL) and associated graphical user interface tools, which enhance end user analysis capabilities. In terms of deployment, this technology is still in its infancy in most organizations. However, it is critical for all business units of the organization, including the clinical laboratory, to participate in the development of this institutional resource because of its long-term value to the organization.

Intranet/Internet Technology

Information access is a major operational issue for health care delivery organizations. The information technology supporting an integrated view of data is still under construction, but information access requirements are immediate. As more physicians and other allied health professionals become members of the integrated delivery system team, the number of sites from which information needs to be accessed greatly increases. A cross-platform (personal computer hardware), easy-to-learn access tool will be required to address this issue. World Wide Web–based Intranet and Internet technology is a leading candidate to fill this void. The majority of ambulatory/hospital information systems vendors are currently porting their software to function in a Web-based environment. The cost of maintaining a private network over broad geographic regions is also driving the switch to Web-based computing to ensure efficient economic operation.

In the short term, Intra/Internet applications are serving the role of information carriers for the integrated delivery system. One example is service information guides (i.e., how specimens are to be collected and processed).

SUMMARY

Organizational and operational change will be the only constant in the health care industry for the near future. Successful clinical laboratories will develop their operation plan in conjunction with the planners of the delivery system from which services are provided. In the age of the integrated delivery system, clinical laboratories that develop information technology strategies, closely linked to a comprehensive clinical information program, will provide a competitive advantage for their organization.

REFERENCES

1. Shortell S: Sustaining a competitive advantage in the 90's. *Hospitals* 1990;64(5):72.
2. Shortell S, Rousseau D, Gillies R: APACHE III study design: analytic plan for evaluation of severity and outcome in intensive care unit patients. Analysis of process. *Crit Care Med* 1989;17(12,Pt2):S213–S216.
3. Dowling AF Jr: Health care information systems architecture of the near future. *J Soc Health Systems* 1989;1(2):77–97.
4. Friedman B, Shortell S: The financial performance of selected investor-owned and not-for-profit system hospitals before and after Medicare prospective payment. *Health Serv Res* 1988;23(2):237–267.
5. Harris CM, Sockolow PS, Petzko DR: Information requirements for an integrated delivery system. MedInfo 95, International Medical Informatics Association, Eighth World Congress of Medical Informatics; 1995.
6. Shulkin DJ, Harris CM: Coordinating initiatives in critical pathways and clinical information systems. *Qual Manage Health Care* 1996;4:37–41.
7. Kelly JT, Swartwout JE: Assisting physicians in decision-making. (Published erratum appears in *Pa Med* 1991;94[10]:42.)
8. Kuperman G, James B, Jacobsen J, Gardner RM: Continuous quality improvement applied to medical care: experiences at LDS hospital. *Med Decis Making* 1991;11(4 Suppl):S60–S65.
9. Conry CM, Pace WD, Main DS: Practice style differences between family physicians and internists. *J Am Board Family Pract* 1991;4(6):399–406.
10. McAlister FA: The potential of critical pathways. *Ann Intern Med* 1996;125(5):427–428.
11. Byrnes J: Lovelace's innovative disease-management program. *Group Pract J* 1996;(July/August):24–28.
12. Tierney WM, Miller ME, Overhage JM, McDonald CJ: Physician inpatient order writing on microcomputer workstations; effects on resource utilization. *JAMA* 1993;269:379–383.
13. Rashke RA, Reilly BM, Guidry JR, Fantana JR, Srinivas S: The weighted basic heparin dosing nomogram compared with standard care nomogram. A randomized controlled trial. *Ann Intern Med* 1993;119(9):874–881.

10
Conclusion

Paul Bozzo

The contents in this book cover subjects that will demand change from day to day. The challenge of cost-effective health care is never ending. Dialogue with clinicians fertilizes new ideas. Uncomfortable interactions occur. You may question your role and ask, "Is this what I really want to do?" The bottom line is a hope that you will continue to make a difference in patient care. We have a budgeted amount of money to spend wisely. Reimbursement policies continue to change, fueled by consumer dissatisfaction with the costs of health care. We should eliminate unnecessary testing: we do not need to do lactic dehydrogenase (LDH) isoenzymes, fecal fats, expensive reflex ordered chromosome tests, and creatine phosphokinases (CPKs) without an elevated total CPK. We need to have a better understanding of finance. We need to use concrete data, not anecdotes in our discussions. We need to look intelligently at point of care testing, robotics, and information technology. A major challenge is to spend enough time looking at these important issues, making them a constructive part of our day. Quality and cost-effectiveness are about a journey, not a destination. This book demonstrates how to venture on that journey, but success is about commitment.

Subject Index

Note: Page numbers followed by f indicate figures; page numbers followed by t indicate tables.